UNMASKED

UNMASKED

*Women Write about Sex and Intimacy
After Fifty*

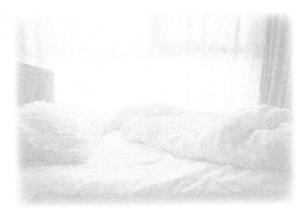

Edited by
Marcia Meier and Kathleen A. Barry, Ph.D.

Weeping Willow Books

Weeping Willow Books
Santa Barbara, California
www.weepingwillowbooks.com

Interior and cover design by Don Mitchell
Cover image by Seeme/Shutterstock.com

ISBN 978-0-9990994-4-5

v1.2

Contents

Pomegranate

Bread

FIGS

INTRODUCTION

WOMEN OVER FIFTY are "the invisible woman" in American culture. In a society that reveres youth—and particularly young, sexy women—women over fifty fade into the shadows. Yet, for many women at mid-life, this is a time of flowering and coming into one's own, sexually and otherwise. Many older women love sex and crave the intimacy it provides. For every story of a harried mother who turns her husband away at night, or the older woman who long ago lost her libido, there are legions of others whose sex drives match those of men.

Women over fifty often are just coming into the most sensual/ sexually pleasurable part of their lives. They've gone through menopause for the most part, and are free of worries about young kids or periods. A Women's Health Initiative study released in 2011 surveyed more than 27,000 U.S. women between fifty and seventy-nine years of age from 1993-98. What it found is that most women in reasonable physical and psychological health enjoyed sex after menopause. In fact, the study found that older women who were in sexual relationships for the most part wanted *more* sex, not less.

The study found that 60 percent of women fifty to fifty-nine were sexually active, that almost 50 percent of women in their sixties

9

were sexually active, and nearly 30 percent of those over seventy were sexually active. Those who were not sexually active listed lack of a partner or a partner with an illness as the main reason.

Sex and intimacy provide many emotional and health benefits, which include:

—Stress reduction. Touching, hugging and sex release oxytocin, the body's natural "feel-good" hormone, which soothes stress and anxiety. One study showed that people who had sex responded better in stressful situations, like public speaking.

—Boosted immunity. "Sexually active people take fewer sick days," says sexual health expert Yvonne K. Fulbright, Ph.D.

—Lowered blood pressure. Research shows it specifically lowers systolic pressure, the top number in blood pressure readings.

—Pain relief. Sex releases a hormone that blocks pain. Researchers have found it effective with leg and muscle aches, menstrual cramps and even headaches.

—Improved sleep. The hormone prolactin is released after sex, which causes feelings of relaxation and sleepiness. Oxytocin, released during orgasm, also promotes sleep.

—Healthier hearts. Sex provides many of the same benefits to your heart as exercise, and keeps levels of estrogen and testosterone in balance, which is important for heart health. Men who have regular sex (at least twice a week) are 45 percent less likely to develop heart disease than men who had sex once a month or less (and masturbation doesn't count).

—Improved bladder control for women. Sex works the muscles of the pelvic floor, which is important to avoid incontinence, which affects about 30 percent of women at some point in their lives.

—An increased sex drive. For women, having sex lubricates the vagina and increases blood flow and elasticity, which makes sex more pleasurable. The more you do it the more you want to do it.

The bottom line: Sex is good for you. So, why is so little attention paid to sex and intimacy among women in later life? Other than a smattering of magazine articles and some academic books, very little has been written about women, sex and intimacy. Oh, there are plenty of how-tos: advice on vaginal dryness and pain during sex and erectile dysfunction. But there is a dearth of work written by women about their sexual experiences after fifty.

So we invited women essayists and poets from around the country to contribute to this anthology, including Bernadette Murphy (*Harley and Me, Embracing Risk on the Road to a More Authentic Life*; *The Tao Gal's Guide to Real Estate*; *Zen and the Art of Knitting*), Diana Raab (*Writing for Bliss, A Seven-Step Program for Telling Your Story and Transforming Your Life*; *Lust*; *Writers on the Edge*), and Ruth Thompson (*Crazing*; *Woman With Crows*; *Here Along Cazenovia Creek*).

We also have poems from extraordinary award-winning writers, including the Pushcart Prize-winning or nominated poets Cathleen Calbert, Liz Rose Dolan, Alexis Rhone Fancher, Irene Fick, Perie Longo, Eileen Malone, Barbara Rockman, Mindela Ruby, Becky Dennison Sakellariou, Carine Topal, Davi Walders, Phyllis Wax, and Brenda Yates.

Unmasked explores everything having to do with sex after fifty for women—the feelings, the romance, the positions, the drawbacks, the orgasms, the risks, the kinky, the sublime, the men and, as the case may be, the women.

For many women, especially those who may have experienced long periods of abstinence for a variety of reasons—widowhood, unsatisfying marriage, impotency of their partners, boredom, loneliness—getting back in the game can be daunting. Until recent years, woman over fifty had few options for meeting eligible men. Online dating has opened up an entirely new arena, and our women talk about how to do it, how not to do it, the men they meet, and the sex. But there are emotional risks inherent. Where does relationship come in? Where does sex end and intimacy begin? And when does intimacy lead to relationship? Can women have sex without emotional involvement, like men do? (The answer is yes, sort of.) Our contributors explore all of this and more.

This collection of essays and poetry is meant to bring sex after fifty for women into the open, to proclaim that it *is* important, it is natural and healthy and, for some women, it is absolutely necessary. E.L. James and her *Fifty Shades of Grey* protagonist Anastasia Steele have nothing on some of our essayists. *Unmasked* will surprise, inform, and—it is hoped—encourage all women of a certain age to (re)discover their sexuality.

—Marcia Meier and Kathleen A. Barry, Ph.D.

HERBS

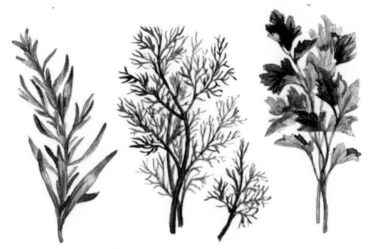

(Enticement)

BERNADETTE MURPHY

ORGASMIC HARLEY, OR WHERE ARE MY BALLS?

IT HAPPENS as I'm astride my Harley traveling across the mighty Mississippi. I'm on a two-week motorcycle road trip from Los Angeles to Milwaukee and back again with my friend Emily, a journey unlike any either of us has taken before, one that's drawing us further outside the suburban mommy realm we've long inhabited and into spaces fresh and unfamiliar. Thanks to a new motorcycle saddle and handlebars, modifications to make my ride more comfortable on this long-haul journey, different parts of my anatomy contact the seat and absorb the pervasive vibrations.

With a row of semis to my right and traffic moving steadily at 80 miles an hour, I feel a tingly sense of buildup. The quivery sensation is exhilarating but totally unsuitable for the occasion. I look over at Emily and the cars streaming past. Is it obvious what's happening?

Slowly, hoping no one notices, I rock my pelvis subtly in time with the vibrations. Mild but gratifying waves of pleasure course through me. This is crazy! Upsurges of delight begin to assemble themselves, adding layer upon layer. I feel my eyes grow wide. Is this

15

really happening? I'm on a bridge traversing the Mississippi in broad daylight surrounded by truckers. My back arches and my hands grip the controls. Waves of euphoria flood my blood with a healthy dose of endorphins. Tingles run along my arms and curl my toes inside heavy leather boots. A shiver makes me sit even taller. Truckers, cowboy-driven pickups, and soccer moms stream past, unaware.

I've gotten away with something amazing. Right here, in public.

I learned to ride a motorcycle two years ago at the age of forty-eight, having watched my father die and my marriage of twenty-five years disintegrate. I was looking for a way to reclaim myself, to step out of the quiet mother-of-three and creative-writing-professor life I'd built.

This was not quite what I had in mind.

And while I've long suspected it might be possible to orgasm on a motorcycle, it has not been my experience, nor have any of the female riders I know ever mentioned it.

Not that I asked.

Discussing sex and its shadowy backroom intricacies is not something I normally indulge in. I believe sex is an ineffable, private experience best left in the realm of the unspoken. But my life is at a crossroads. It's asking me to delve into the sphere of the tacit and give voice to what has previously been unsaid, to open myself up to new paradigms, to be vulnerable and gutsy and real. Because, really: what will my life hold now that the old blueprint of getting married, having kids, and building a home life together no longer applies? What am I moving toward, single at fifty?

After the orgasm subsides, I wonder if I should say anything to Emily. Perhaps I've unknowingly morphed into some kind of lone cougar. Anything is possible. I might be picking up thirty-year-olds before this trip is over.

The truth is, sex has been on my mind a lot since my marriage ended, certainly a lot more than I expected. Just a few weeks ago I purchased condoms, something I've never done. There is no man, active or fanciful, in my life. Still, the condoms are a talisman, giving me assurance that I won't be sexless the rest of my days. I am waking up from a deep narcolepsy to find myself in a new and unfamiliar land, utterly flummoxed to be here.

I am celibate for the first time in my adult life.

We stop at a motel for the night. When Emily is in the shower, I Google: "orgasm on motorcycle?" One woman's comment cracks me up: "Are you kidding? All the bashing around on my lady parts. No way!"

A guy answers the question: "My last wife used to get off on the Harley vibration, but it was such a pain getting the 650-pound bike into the bed and then washing the oil and chain lube out of the sheets that we only did it that way a few times." One woman claims the experience of riding a motorcycle with Ben Wa balls is delicious, causing waves of orgasms to keep her company.

I realize I have taken sex far too seriously my entire life. While most of my friends were busy exploring their nascent sexuality as twenty-somethings, I was married and having kids. Maybe it's time for some exploration. And really, let's face it: If not now, when?

I find a website for a store in Albuquerque, where we'll be in a few days. The shop claims it's a guilt-free, shame-free environment. I finally screw up my courage and approach Emily.

"So, there's this place in Albuquerque." I lay out the whole story: the orgasm on the Mississippi (which, disappointingly, has not occurred since), plus what I've learned on the Internet.

She laughs. "This could be interesting."

We find the sex shop midday, a florid storefront in a sketchy neighborhood. I'd been hoping it might be more inviting. I explain my mission to the helpful young woman working there. She goes through the various options and convinces me that the best approach is a single silicone ball the size of a jawbreaker. It's a good introductory choice. "If nothing else, you'll improve your pelvic floor muscles by doing Kegel contractions."

I step into the bathroom and put the ball inside. At my insistence, Emily also buys one but decides to wait to experiment.

As I ride, I keep waiting to feel the first hint of that distinctive tingle. Nothing. It's as exciting as having inserted a tampon.

Eventually, I figure I may as well do some Kegel exercises. At least *some* good will come of all this.

When we stop for gas, Emily comes over. "Well?"

"Utterly underwhelming."

The next leg of our journey is memorable for two reasons. The first is the remarkable scenery as we parallel the New Mexico-Arizona border. It's desert-like, with rolling hills that approach and recede, filling my eyes with subtle desert hues against a brilliant cerulean sky. The second is that all those Kegels must have jumpstarted the Ben-Wa ball. Over a distance of about 100 miles, I experience a dozen gentle, rolling orgasms and am kept in a state of heightened arousal. They're not the slam-bang magnitude of orgasm that leaves me limp and speechless, but subtle and enchanting and send shivers up my back.

It's inappropriate as hell. But sometimes life asks us to let go and just live.

When we next stop for gas, I grab Emily by the arm and look deep into her eyes. "You. Must. Try. This."

She laughs. "I knew something was going on. You kept speeding up, and then for no reason, slowing way down. Your driving was really erratic. Please don't do this when we get back to LA," she warns. "With traffic, you'll be asking for an accident."

"But really, Emily, you've got to experience this!"

She waves me off.

I've spent my entire life being appropriate, seemly, correct, and reliable. I've been invested and loving as a mom, loyal as a wife, rousing as a professor, dutiful as a daughter, steadfast as a friend. At this time in my life, it's not about filling any of those roles. Appropriateness, I decide, is way overrated. It's my turn to let loose.

"Besides," she demurs, climbing back on her bike. "One of us needs to be the designated driver."

She's right, of course. But at least for today, it's not going to be me.

MAYA SHAW GALE

PERSEPHONE REVEALED

First of all, let it be known—
I hate pomegranates
those gritty little pellets
coated in gelatinous red slime
that mythology has come to blame
for my descent into the underground.
Hell no! Not one of those nasty seeds
ever touched *my* lips.
That was just a ruse
to convince my mother that I stayed against my will.
The truth is I'm a Scorpio, born to be wild
and magnetized to the shadow like a bat to its cave.
I lost my virginity long before
Hades got his big hairy hands on me,
but I never had hotter, juicier, yoni-throbbing sex
than I had with him. All those horny shepherds
that came before were mere boys playing at passion
and my true womanhood was never
going to be awakened by such wimps.
So all you fools and fiction lovers
who are feeling sorry for me
being trapped down here in the bowels of the Earth
for six months every year, you can
shed all the sympathy tears you want.
But if I had my druthers, I'd never have to pop up
like that sappy little crocus in spring,
wearing my virginal whites and pretending relief
as I rush into Demeter's smotherly arms.

I'd be staying right where I am,
wrapped in Hades' muscular embrace,
wearing my black lace negligee
and screwing my blissful brains out
all year long!

CATHARINE BRAMKAMP

IN THE PRADO

I live
He smiled
On the second floor
On the Calle Canaletto de Gracio
Rolling the R relishing
The feel of the name between his lips

She shifted her bag
Squirted another measure of
Hand sanitizer

I live in the US on S. 45th St
Not pronouncing the long E
It took too long

His Greco eyes slowed her
She took his hand—forgetting
To clean

Come I can make for you
An afternoon that will last
Till the death of summer

LOLA FONTAY

My First "Date" at Sixty-One

FRENCH WRITER AND NOBEL PEACE PRIZE WINNER Andre Gide says that one does not discover new lands without consenting to lose sight of the shore for a very long time. My experience as a widow in the unfamiliar waters known as online dating has been similar to Gide's perspective.

Early on in the journey, I unknowingly agreed to lose sight of the familiar shore of my life and set sail on unfamiliar seas heading toward unknown lands. I am sixty-one-years-old and single for the first time in twenty-six years after losing my husband and soul mate to a sudden heart attack three years ago. Granted, I had a full love life as a single woman during the 1970s and '80s. However, the journey as an older woman who has known one lover for a quarter of a century is quite different from that of a twenty- to thirty-year-old dating several men at one time while waiting for the "love of her life" to arrive.

I was terrified filling out the required information on the first website I joined. My niece and nephew graciously offered direction and wording as I wrote my profile. I was asked to provide personal data about my favorite books, music, and movies, queried about my most enjoyable activities, and encouraged to describe my ideal date (do they mean "mate" I wondered?). I was tentative in my answers—offering very little information about myself—thinking "it's none of their business," which is not the best attitude to adopt as one is becoming a player in the online dating scene! Since then I have become more brazen and now regularly surf five different dating sites. I have been on a couple dozen "dates" and overall, I have found the experience poignant, challenging, and an uncomfortable yet delicious adventure. I would say for the most part that the men I have met have been great guys—each bringing something new to my expanding resume as an online aficionado, a sensuous older woman, and an overall charming individual to get to know.

My first date was with DH, who was an intriguing sixty-two-year-old man with whom I felt an instant rapport when we spoke by phone. He was articulate, bright, a great conversationalist, and we shared many interests. We decided to set up a date to meet at a restaurant a few days later. Immediately upon hanging up, I scoured the web and gratefully learned that the narrative he offered during our phone conversation matched what I found from the various online sources I checked. I told many friends about my pending first date and they cheered me on. I also set up safety precautions with one of my good friends—I would text her from the restaurant bathroom if I was uncomfortable. I also promised that I would text her when I returned home from the date.

As I got ready, I felt the giddy excitement of a twenty-something. I carefully applied my new makeup, dressed myself in an outfit that conveyed class and yet was sexy. It was also a black outfit—more slimming you know! I am voluptuous and athletic ... code on online dating sites that I am not thin, but not grossly "overweight." When I decided I was ready to go, I spritzed myself with my favorite Chanel perfume, took one last look in the mirror, and walked out the door—feeling peculiar, unfamiliar with the experience, missing my husband, and yet determined to start the journey of a thousand miles—which starts with a single step, right? When I arrived at the restaurant, a bottle of white wine awaited me at the hostess desk. I thought it was DH who was surprising me before I even arrived at the table.

"Wow, what a guy!" I thought. I proudly carried the bottle as I followed the hostess to the table where DH was waiting for me. When I saw him I was pleased—I liked his face and smile. His clothes were neat, clean, and I liked the colors he chose. I was relieved that he looked normal. I asked about the wine and he clarified that it was not his doing. I was mildly disappointed and embarrassed that I thought he did such a wonderful thing like this (something my late husband would have done!). I searched for a card and found one attached to the side. It was from my trainer, who had left the bottle for me as a congrats. The card stated: "You go girl, have fun, drink up, we will work off the calories tomorrow!"

Dinner went smoothly—he was funny and delightful. He finished what I didn't eat from my dinner and that felt remarkably comforting and pleasant. We learned from our discussions that we had friends in common. The evening went by quickly and I did not want it to end. Despite the "experts" (as well as my close friends) who tell newbies to not invite anyone back to your place, I decided that I would extend an invitation since we *did* have mutual friends in common. Before we left the comforts of the restaurant booth we had shared for over three hours, I was emphatic in letting him know that I live in a gated community, with a guard, and that I would tell the guard that he would be allowed to follow me in. I think he got the message that he could not assault me in my home. We walked to our cars and I liked how it felt to have the strong arm of a man encircling me once again. He made it past the guard, we parked our cars, and walked hand-in-hand up to my oceanfront condo.

He was dumfounded by where I lived and I could sense he was a bit impressed. We sat on the couch and he put his arm around me and we kissed. I was aware of feeling numb from the neck down—I had not kissed anyone in three years. Our kissing moved to the preliminary stages that would be expected of two people who found one another attractive … French kissing, necking, petting … nothing more—*until* I became aware that DH was unzipping his pants. I stopped him and said things were not going *that* far, and he laughed. He proceeded to pull out his penis and masturbate in front of me. I was stunned and intrigued at the same time. I had not been prepared for *that*, thinking he presumed we would move right into intercourse. With my head on his shoulder and my eyes surveying the "goods" that he had to offer (I was pleased by what I saw), and in a somewhat betwixt and between state of mind, I watched him finish the job in a remarkably short period of time.

Coming back to real time and remembering where I was, I saw that DH had come all over himself and did not have a cloth handkerchief in his pocket, but why would he? Men have not carried cloth handkerchiefs in fifty-plus years! I bolted to the kitchen and gathered several pieces of tissue from the holder on the counter. I handed them to him and he cleaned the thick white liquid off himself and placed the "goods" back in his pants. You might wonder what two people in this situation might talk about in the not-so-afterglow of the moment.

I found out there is *nothing* to talk about after a man I have known for approximately three and a half hours masturbates in front of me, in my living room, with my three cats sitting on a nearby ottoman watching us. I was not angry with him; I was more shocked and dumbfounded by his action and my inaction.

I walked him to his car and noticed it was a warm and balmy central California coast winter evening. The ocean sounds were soothing and melodic. I kissed him goodbye and we agreed to meet again later in the week. Back in my home, I went to the living room and then I felt angry. I spotted a familiar clump of white tissue on the table next to where DH sat. He left the "seeds" of his efforts on my glass-covered skirted table—the one that had been in my husband's den in the larger home I sold after his death. I threw the pile of tissues away and felt dirtied and saddened. When I got into bed, I saw that my friend had sent me a text an hour earlier. She was wondering where I was…it was midnight and my date started at 7 p.m. I could not tell her for several weeks what had happened. I felt embarrassed because I had acted impulsively and felt cheapened by the experience.

I texted DH the next day and described my reactions. He apologized and wanted to speak by phone. He also wanted to get together again. I declined both requests.

Even though my first date experience was uncomfortable, I learned from it. I realized how I am still influenced by patriarchal tenets that dictate how "good girls" need to behave and simultaneously give permission to "bad boys" of any age to go for what they want. I decided to challenge these double standards and go for the gusto with each of the men I meet. I have learned that women and men can have fun at any age. At this point of my life, I have paid my social/cultural dues and am fully planning on sharing intellectual, physical, and sexual passion with men who have the "right stuff" that I require in a relationship.

First of all, they must want to meet a woman like me, one who is smart, well-educated, tender, pretty, sexy, and voluptuous. Moreover, a woman who is ever the wiser from what I now refer to as the "DH" litmus test.

SARAH BROWN WEITZMAN

AFTER READING FIFTY SHADES AT SEVENTY-FIVE

The clever sign, FORePLAY, drew me in
to wander self-consciously
among displays of dildos,
fleshlike latex, Pepto-Bismol-pink
hard plastic blacks, never red.

More familiar among
condoms. But a rising
fever in the S&M section
whips, crops, blindfolds and
the terrible softness of velvet
wrist cuffs & collars.

Recognizing in a sudden rush
why, inflamed by desire,
the ancient martyrs
had believed heaven
could be gained in a fire.

LISA MAE DeMASI

THE KICKASS FORMULA THAT RESTORED MY LIBIDO AT FIFTY

"The Female Orgasm. The Big O. That elusive, reclusive Loch Ness of the labia. Does it prove the existence of God, or just His twisted sense of humor?"
— Kirstie Collins Brote, *Beware of Love in Technicolor*

THROUGH THE CLOSED LIDS OF MY EYES, I feel the morning sunlight streaming in.

Hey, it's the weekend.

I take inventory of my brain for traces of a hangover.

We're in the clear.

And then I check for any activity that might be stirring in the netherworld between my legs, which has, of late, been about as playful as a schoolmarm.

Nothing.

I can hear Chris breathing beside me. Sweet beautiful man, and yet for weeks now no amount of touching or stroking or licking on his part can bring back the phenomenon of rapture, nothing eases our hearty pursuit of it. Chris has tried; I've grimaced.

Sex-wise, everything was going great until I hit fifty. Because it had been so easy before, I couldn't understand why climaxing had become like trudging up Mount Washington with a dead body strapped to my back.

A quick Google search advised me to: "Get a pedicure, touch up your roots, spritz on your favorite perfume, get some exercise, schedule your sex, add a toy or two, try porn..."

Nothing.

But lately I've wondered if this was about something that KY Jelly can't fix.

Hidden in my bedside drawer are sweet almond and rose oil and some ylang ylang I got at the organic food store. These oils are aphrodisiacs, but they are also antidepressants, hypotensives, nervines, and sedatives, and while I want that man sleeping beside me to slip inside and have a go, there's also a reason I want the regular, easy cures to work.

I don't want to acknowledge the changes going on in my fifty-year-old body, the fact that I am no longer wet at the drop of a man's hand feels like a failure somehow.

And, because I feel like a failure, I've been avoiding my body and therefore my self-Reiki practice. Reiki, a wild healing energy we can apply to ourselves, seeks out what's maligned and out of whack in the body—blocks to creativity, depression, grief. It's a catalyst to deepening spirituality that can offer glimpses of the divine.

On this Saturday morning with the aromatherapy hidden in my bedside table, I think: And isn't sex divine?

With self-Reiki, you put your hands on yourself (absolutely anywhere, it really doesn't matter...your arm, your belly) and bring your life force through your hands and into the body.

So, on this light-filled Saturday morning, because I am dying (literally) to be with the guy I used to crave, because last night during a scotch-induced haze I fell asleep while he was saying, "How about this?" and I was saying, "Nothing," I put my hands on my abdomen and start.

My hands get warm, and I feel a deep sense of relaxation, not sleep but something wider, more alive.

That energy, whatever it is, doesn't care whether you can have sex or not, how old you are, if you are getting a pudge around your middle, how many wrinkles have settled around your eyes.

Time slips away, I slip away, all that remains is blissed-out peace. Like drinking a martini—without the edge.

When I finish, I eyeball Chris. His eyes are half-mast, he's styling an alfalfa hairdo, an imprint from a crease in his pillowcase runs across the right side of his face.

Not exactly a turn-on, but I don't care. "Let's give it a go," I say.

Being a man in love (if he's not too far under the influence of scotch), Chris is always ready to give it a go.

With a blind hand, I pull the end table drawer open and fumble for oil I concocted from the health food store.

Forget the sticky KY goop, this stuff glides like heaven.

Chris gets his hands on the love rub, goes about the business of inducing the hopeful rapture amid my numb equipment.

I anticipate the onslaught of banter that has ensued for the past few months like doc to patient:

"Here?"

"No."

"How about here?"

"Nothing."

Those myriad times when I can no longer tell if his are the hands of a green gynecologist or a prospective cow buyer at auction.

But today something whispers: *Hang in, be still.*

Be still?

Stop trying so hard; relax. Look, there, out into the horizon.

That little voice sounds suspiciously like my intuition. I don't hear it very often, mostly because I'm too busy listening to the voices saying I'm not supple enough, pretty enough, I'm past my prime...

The horizon? I ask it.

Behind your eyes.

There's a horizon in my head?

Just close your eyes.

In my head, a cumulonimbus cloud appears in the distance, rolling with great billows of white particles.

The atmosphere changes.

And the change is charged.

"Here?" asks Chris.

Humidity—wet blanket type—sweeps in.

"Lisa?"

The storm hits.

A jagged line of electricity streaks across the room and touches my numb equipment. A lively spark ignites. Eyes squeezed closed, my heart pounds, I begin to sweat, my breath comes in short gasps. The spark ignites into flame, deep inside a pinch expands like fire to paper. I'm sucked into a trippy spiraling vortex.

The rapture fills me—a delicious swell that comes from the bottom of the ocean, too big to be experienced for but a moment or two.

The wave recedes, leaving me pie-eyed, legs in rigor, fists clenched tight.

I look to Chris, who is hovering over me, his expression one of delight, the crease from the pillowcase stretched thin against the smiling muscles of his cheek. Given that he has a technical mind and has a limited repertoire of reactions, it's rather comical.

"The self-Reiki," I say, "the essential oils." I catch wind of my torso. It's charred in places and emits wisps of smoke.

We may have a formula to bring about a bit of the ol' spark.

As the blood begins to seep back into my flesh, I let out a laugh— ribald, raucous. Besides having a great partner who will push and prod without feeling like a jackass, and will let you get as woo-woo as you want in the sack, I no longer feel old. Sex can last until ninety. We just need to nurture ourselves in order to feel sparked about anything, including our libido.

And, in order to feel the wonders of the Universe, we need to let go and let god, whatever the hell your definition of god is, to be a part of it.

PHYLLIS WAX

THE WIDOW REVIVES

The earth thaws,
sucks at my boots.
Sap's oozing.
The mild air fluffs my heart.

I find myself moving the ring
to my right hand,
eying male faces.

The indolence of winter
drops away. Birds gather twigs
and build, start over each day.
Buds loosen, dogs race
and play. I think I'll shave my legs.

ANGELA LOCKE

CHRISTINE

I'D BEEN AWAY FROM WORK for a few years, and was coming back as a new coordinator. I would have some authority this time around, though not much. Enough to have to lead meetings, which is where I saw her. Seventy people, maybe eighty, were in the audience, some I knew from the previous years, many I didn't. Glancing over the seated people, waving hello to my old co-workers, some coming up to hug me: that's when I saw her. I stopped; as the cliché goes, the old heart skipped a beat; I actually wondered for a second if this is why I'd been "led" to come back to something I'd left. I also had time to wonder if she was a lesbian—no use going crazy if she wasn't—and if she had a partner. When she looked up from what she was doing and looked right at me, I thought of the scene in "West Side Story" where Tony and Maria see each other across the room.

Did that date me just now, the "West Side Story" reference? Was I thirteen when I saw this woman, like Shakespeare's Juliet when she met Romeo? Was I nineteen, the age when I fell for just about anyone who paid attention to me?

No. I was fifty-eight; she was sixty-two.

Young people think they invented sex. I remember in the early seventies when a guy pressuring me to have sex said: "Sex is recreation now. Sex is not what your parents did. Sex is fun and everyone is doing it with everyone else. It's like a damn good game of tennis."

What strikes me about that statement, other than the lame come-on, are the two implications: 1. Our parents did not have fun, and 2. Saying sex is what our parents "did" implies that their sex is in the past tense, that they "did" it to conceive their children (us), and then it was over. My parents would have been in their fifties at the time of my friend's unsuccessful attempt to get me into bed. Maybe it's because as their children we can't imagine our parents doing the things that thrill *us* out of our minds. Maybe not the prettiest picture to think of those stern, old-fashioned authority figures with their *bodies* (oh god, even that image…) in various stages of undress and compromise.

I did meet the woman in the first paragraph and, yes, we had some fun. We used to laugh about the younger people around, in a café or in a restaurant, holding hands or kissing across the table. "They only see a couple of old ladies," one of us said once. "If they only knew!"

If young people and the culture-at-large draw conclusions about older people not having or loving sex, the judgment might be harsher upon women. You sometimes hear someone say, "He's sixty years old and he has a new wife and a baby!" But you don't hear people say, "She's shacking up with a thirty-year-old. Lucky guy!"

And if the opinion is erroneous about older women, it might be doubly so for older lesbians. Many heterosexual people have wondered, "But what do they *do?*"

I've never been a kiss-and-tell kind of girl. I never shared intimate information with my girlfriends the way some girls did. They would sit around and talk details, and I mean details: exactly what he did, how long it took, where he touched, where she touched, what it looked like. Whether it's my Presbyterian upbringing or a chromosome for a strict personal privacy code, I don't get into specifics. But I will say this: After forty years of having and liking sex, there was no loss of anything, no lack, no hesitation, no doctors needed, no ointments, no adaptations. Not that there is anything wrong with doctors, ointments or adaptations. Those are not weaknesses; those are figuring out how to get, and give, pleasure, and they have their place. But in our case—two old ladies others may have thought did nothing but hang around the house baking cookies for grandchildren, crocheting toilet paper covers, and talking about our African violets—no.

We were very busy, in bed, in hotel rooms, on the sofa, on the massage table, and in bed again. Very busy having fun.

BAMBI BARKER

BAMBI READS SYDNEY SHELDON

With Hermès scarves
she ties each of his hands
to a hotel dresser leg

Straddles his otherwise unembellished
body while she reads a section
from *The Other Side of Midnight*

Where another *she* dumps
a bucket of champagne ice
on another *he's* hard act to follow

Not for her though
As she leaves the door wide open
to go find an ice machine

DEBBIE BROSTEN

THE AGE OF AMBIVALENCE

A FRIEND I HAVEN'T SPOKEN WITH in months calls to catch up. She gushes about her new grandson. We talk about her trip to Portugal, mine to Japan. She brings me up to date on the women in the book club I helped form years ago when I lived in their town. I hear about the new quilt she is working on. She asks how my writing groups are going. Then, she mentions the charming new man in her life. She is a good friend, a good person, and I wish I could report that my initial reaction was joy, but alas, I'm not that altruistic. I throw a silent self-pity party before mirroring her enthusiasm for the new turn in her life. After disconnecting, I reflect on my own life. I am painfully aware no man, charming or otherwise, is ringing my bell. Realizing it is up to me, I join a dating site.

I put myself out there even though I am no longer young or supple. My silver hair, even though it is long and silky, allows for no pretense. Nor does my increasingly crêpey skin. I compose an online profile highlighting my love of travel and my sense of humor. I scan my photos for ones that don't make me cringe, and submit it all. Before I'm even approved I type in the parameters of the man I am seeking and scroll through dozens of pictures. Instinctively I sort them in my head; maybes, no-ways and occasional ahhhs. The no-ways make up the biggest category: bearded men who could be replacements on "Duck Dynasty," the shirtless who mistakenly think that exposing their aging skin is a good idea, the tragic spellers, the seriously young searching for a sugar mama, and the ones whose profiles contain not a hint of humor or personality. The maybes are those who sparked a second look due to travel or cute dog photos, an interesting resume, or something that comes through as real. Most important, these men use words well and seduce me with clever or funny lines. The ahhhs are the too handsome, too rich, and probably too self-absorbed, but nonetheless cause wild fantasies to bloom.

Soon my computer dings, alerting me to incoming messages. I log onto the site. Loverboy likes my photo. I don't like his scraggly beard almost as much as I disdain his screen name. I delete that email. I'mYourDreamGuy is an admirable wordsmith despite his penchant for cheesy screen names. He is also a professor at the local university, so I respond to him. We exchange flirty quips and decide to meet for dinner. He is better looking than his photo. Or maybe it's the tweed jacket he's wearing with his comfortable jeans; a look I've always found alluring. We decide on sushi. Our conversation covers his love of music and my enthusiastic reaction to Bellingham, where I resettled a year ago. He doesn't suggest another meeting and neither do I, although to be honest, I wouldn't have minded investing a bit more time and energy into a possible relationship. I thanked him for dinner and moved on, feeling discouraged.

Back to the site. I email someone who seems interesting based on what he has posted. I tell him his dog is a winner. We meet for coffee. At least he's drinking a latte, while I sip my Earl Grey tea. He tells me he enjoys cooking and suggests we do it together sometime. I would prefer to know him better before inviting him to my apartment or showing up at his house, so we arrange a couple more dates, a dinner, a movie.

He offers to bring the ingredients for a menu of my choice. On a pre-arranged evening, we self-consciously bump around my small kitchen as he dices garlic, onions and ginger, and I stir broth into the brewing risotto. The bottle of pinot noir he uncorked quickly empties as dinner and conversation progress. A reach around into drawers or cabinets provides the opportunity for a hand to linger on a waist or shoulder, until finally an embrace refuses to back off. We settle into a kiss. Insistent risotto bubbles us apart. Smiles linger.

"Are you having fun?" he asks. I smile my response as we return to the chopping and stirring. Yet as the shrimp sears, the asparagus roasts golden, I worry. "Too much? Too soon?" We transfer the creamy mushroom risotto to our earthenware plates, add the shrimp and asparagus and sit together at the round table. Appreciative sighs of contentment rise unbidden as we congratulate ourselves on our joint effort.

Dinner complete, I rise to clear the plates. "I can help," he offers. "No need," I answer. "Are you kicking me out or can I stay the evening?" he asks as he rises. I catch the hitch in my step before he notices, although he might have seen my shoulders sag. "No," I respond, wondering how the options have so quickly whittled down to unacceptable alternatives. "Too soon" plays through my head. "I'm not sure I like you that much," I think, but don't say.

Aren't we too old for indiscriminate sex with body parts that no longer always comply with our desires? With bodies we are no longer anxious to share in the light? "How about if we get to know each other first?" I counter. The next day he sends an email, asks if we can do it again. Life interrupts that next date as his daughter and her family come for a visit. While they are here, I leave for a visit with my mother back East. A friend comes for the weekend when I return. I have heard nothing from my cooking partner since his family arrived. After my friend leaves, I text, suggesting we get together. I quickly receive a response. Seems he enjoyed meeting me, I'm a great woman, BUT he met someone else. Good luck with my search, he says. It's a toss-up whether I'm disappointed or relieved. Being dumped, even if you aren't all that interested, still stings.

Back to the site. JustTHEOneForYou has messaged me, says he would like to get together for lunch. Lunch has morphed into happy hour by the time details are finalized. A glass of rich Syrah clones itself into a second as we trade stories, a commodity easily shared over drinks and a plate of pan-fried oysters. Soon not just his head and upper torso are leaning into the table, but his hand tests the waters too. He grasps my fingers, quickly releasing them while he searches my face for approval. My reaction is ambivalent. I am not particularly attracted to this man, but it feels wonderful to be touched again.

The need to be seen, to be appreciated, clouds my judgment. I neither encourage this contact, nor pull away. This need harkens back to the hole left in childhood when our mothers were too busy to respond to our desires the moment they arose. "Change me, feed me, hold me. I'm uncomfortable. Fix it!" That small gash deepens over time, accentuated by divorce and break–ups. These repeated experiences gouge out more of our self-worth. Regardless of intentions, we are left with an achy wound.

So my fingers reach back as he pronounces me prettier than my photo. On their own they seek the warmth, the acceptance he is offering. He misreads my smile born of discomfort as something more than was intended. The goodbye kiss, a foregone conclusion given my acceptance of his overtures, is not entirely unwelcome. My reaction to it leaves me suspicious of my intentions as well. After all, I put myself out there, advertised on a dating site, proclaimed to the world that I was lacking.

That night he sends a text, informs me where he will be at brunch the next day. He tells me (tells, not asks) to meet him. I decline knowing we have nothing in common. He makes no further contact. This time I am relieved.

As I again scan profiles I question my need to connect. I wonder if I truly believe I am lacking or if I have merely fallen victim to society's dictates. Everywhere there are couples, families. I watch "House Hunters International," indulging my traveler's lust. I sift the couples' experiences into my single one. I am very familiar with foreign travel, and solo travel, yet relocating as a single inhibits the choices I find acceptable. The burdens, as well the opportunities, are greater. While I have many single friends, there is no mistaking that we are a minority. The Great American Dream is built around the happiness found in couple hood. Madison Avenue pastes this message on billboards, in magazines and it naturally spills out into TV and the movies.

I think of my cousin who has been divorced for over twenty years. In all that time she has only involved herself in one short relationship. She busies herself with her children, her grandchildren, her friends, her work. She says she doesn't have time or energy for more. I find myself pitying her. Unlike her, I am not ready to give up the companionship or the sex. I miss the intimacy, the physical release, feeling desirable.

Occasionally I still attract men and it seems to catch me by surprise. Last year I was on Isla Mujeres in Mexico. I had gone by myself, but quickly met up with a couple of fun women. They had been on the island for weeks and knew a group of people. When one of their friends, a younger man, came on to me, I was oblivious until he maneuvered me into a lone walk back to my hotel. It wasn't until his lips met mine that I caught on. Thinking what happens on the island, stays on the island, I indulged. Being pursued by a man I found intriguing and attractive was akin to a dip in the proverbial fountain of youth.

A few months ago I was on a day trip with a friend in the local mountains where I met an attractive man around my age. We exchanged information. That evening I received a clever text, but I was leaving town the next day. When I returned, he was on the way to Oregon to attend to his ailing father. The weeks since we met have lengthened. Sporadically one or the other of us suggests a meet-up. Responses are quick in coming, yet memories of what we look like fade as our calendars conflict. Still the exhilaration of being noticed was, well, exhilarating.

My ex comes for a short visit. We indulge in the good parts of our relationship, the laughter, the affection, the sex, ignoring the jabs that caused hurt feelings when we were focused on making the other into our perfect mate. I know he will never take better care of himself or stop making sarcastic remarks. He knows I will never let him off the hook. Understanding there is no future frees us to enjoy each other as we did when we first met. We discuss our attempts at finding love, companionship. He tells me these other men don't know what they are missing. I want to believe him. For now, I stop expecting my phone to ring or ding. I go about my life doing things that make me happy. I scan new situations for possibilities. I contemplate spending the rest of my life alone. Or as alone as my circle of friends allows me to be. I tell myself it is enough. Sometimes I choose to believe it.

RUTH THOMPSON

SECOND CHILDHOOD

For Lucille Clifton

Bless Lucille's big hips!
And bless my own free-at-last hips!
Here they are dawdling
and not worrying one
bit about where they are
in relation
to anyone else.

You can look at me or not.
I am not saying anything personal anymore.

I am saying hips breasts belly legs feet
roots branches and big thick trunk
tides
sunrises
monkeys lithe and witty in the dawn trees
tigers shaking out oiled stripes of sun and shadow—

I say you can look at me or not.
I am busy dancing—
freckled
and fond
and fat as the fat old sun.

Angela M. Franklin

Straight with No Chaser

Initially, I didn't think I'd have much to say about sex after fifty because I'm not sexually active and haven't been for some time.

Being sexually active doesn't define my womanhood or my perception of myself as a desirable woman. One of the reasons I haven't been engaging in the bedroom boogie isn't because I can't get a date or can't attract the opposite sex. That's not the case. I've chosen celibacy because of my faith and religious beliefs, so I don't feel like I'm missing out on anything I haven't done before.

I know I can be sexually aroused; I have feelings just like the next warm-blooded human being. At sixty-two years young, all of my parts are in good working order, and I am still attractive and sexy. I tend to attract younger men, which amuses me because I'm not looking to tuck anyone in at night.

Temptation had potential to arm wrestle me into the bedroom if it weren't for my fear of being disappointed by someone in my age group being unable to perform well or meet my sexual needs. I'd rather stay alone than be aggravated. I've heard the stories of men lasting only two or three minutes, and then, poof—they collapse like a three-legged chair. I'm sure challenges of sicknesses and disease impact a man's virility in such cases. Erectile dysfunction can be downright disappointing for both parties involved in the sex act. If that weren't true, sexual performance drugs wouldn't be in demand.

Once, I was dating a mature man with great sex appeal. He smelled delicious and had a touch that made me melt like butter on a hot skillet. Luke had it going on with his full lips that felt like I was kissing rose petals. Other women wanted him and were always in his face, but he was after me. I wasn't even attracted to him initially because we were friends with common interests and goals. I was someplace else mentally as I was in the throes of graduate classes after nearly twenty-five years away from college. I even told him I wasn't feeling the intimate relationship thing.

Being the man he was, he set out to conquer my notion of singlehood. One day, I was visiting him and he made a move by kissing me when I was distracted. At first, I thought hmmm, *what, but, but, but? Well, all righty then. What else are you working with?* His lips were soft and inviting, so I kissed him back eagerly, to my utter surprise. It was like a lit match on the drought-stricken bed of the Angeles Forest. I hadn't been involved with anyone in so long I'd forgotten what a kiss felt like. His tongue became an independent crown fire that leaped over the trees of my religious resistance and combusted areas long drenched with cold water piety, or so I thought. We kissed with such passion that my lips hurt for days after that initial encounter. Can a woman take fire in her bosom and not be ignited?

We began dating and would have some kiss and petting fests like two starving teenagers. He vowed to kiss me at least 100 times each time we got together. I'd close my eyes and lose count after juicy kisses wet areas along my jawline, shoulder blades and nipples. Mentally, I'd wind up on some uncharted oasis and lose myself in the moment, ignoring the voices of resistance telling me what I shouldn't be doing. I closed my eyes to lips that forged new paths on the mountaintops and valleys on my body.

I'd forgotten what it felt like for a man to hold and caress me. Sometimes, I would just lie nestled in the arms of his Hugo Boss content like a baby after depleting an engorged breast. I called him my sure-hand Luke. He knew how to hold and caress me like I was a prized piece of pottery recently excavated from a sacred archeological site. This man had serious moves! Most of all, he made me feel desirable and beautiful despite middle-aged weight gain and other demerits of aging. Luke's tenderness caused me to carry myself with greater confidence because of all the doting attention he lavished on me.

I wasn't a sixteen-year-old girl with raging hormones anymore, so I was willing to make him, and me, wait. I needed to get to know Luke on a personal level. I called it allowing a buildup, if you will, of excitement for the final act of sexual intimacy. Up to that point, my built-in stop clock would keep me in check just before things went further than I desired.

One particular evening after a great meal he prepared and good wine, we sat kissing and fishing areas of ourselves stiffened with desire, while the television watched us. After turning the room into a sauna with our rising temperatures and racing heartbeats, he asked if I was ready to go to the next level. He was ready to launch into the deep.

"Can I put it in?" he asked, his voice low like distant thunder before the clap.

"What?" I asked coyly, like I hadn't heard him. He went an octave lower, Barry White-ish.

"You know, can I get it in? I want to feel all of you around me, girl."

"Uh, the question is can *you* handle me around you?"

"Let's give it a try and see where it goes."

Now, see, that's when the mental warning bells went off. I'm thinking, *What? I don't think you know if you can toe the line. 'Let's see where it goes' didn't sound too certain.* What he was really saying was he didn't know how *long* he could last during the act. I could tell because we had been fooling around one day, and he lay on top of me kissing and it felt like I was laying under three sacks of wet cement. I thought to myself, he didn't know that he shouldn't put all of his weight of me. I felt like I was being smothered. I could barely breathe.

Luke's response made me recall Raelene's sexual insights as a woman of sixty-one. "I typically date men around my same age. But I don't like old men. At this stage of the game, I'm not going to date someone sixty-nine or older. That is old to me. I'll date someone a couple of years older than me, but that's about it. I will not date someone taking Viagra or any other enhancer. My man doesn't need Viagra," my attractive and stylishly dressed grandmother friend explained.

I asked her why she wouldn't date a man who needed to take sexual performance drugs for erectile dysfunction if he needed help. Raelene's sigh signaled what I should have been able to figure out. "You've heard those commercials. Listen to the warnings about possible side effects. ...*if you have an erection lasting more than four hours...seek medical attention immediately...*HA! Lasting four hours? Four hours? Hmmm, whatever you're going to do with *that* erection is not going to include me. I know of a man who had to go to the emergency room because he was one of those users that had a four-hour erection. Don't ask me how he came back to normal because I changed the subject. He had nerve to want to date me. I told him he was geographically unattractive (he lived over 100 miles away)."

Raelene added: "My stuff is natural. I would fear him having a heart attack (if he takes sex enhancers). I don't want anyone dying on me. You know what they say about dead weight. I may not be able to remove him and he might end up suffocating me to death." She was quite serious. I asked her, what if her man could no longer perform? She winked and said, "Well, if he can't cut the mustard, he can always lick the jar."

I thought about Raelene's fears and had a fleeting "what if" moment. I was unsure of Luke's unsureness. At that moment I was sort of turned off a little and knew there was no way I could possibly allow him to *get it in* as he put it. But, we continued kissing and touching. I had no need for a lubricant, despite being several years into menopause. I was aroused but not enough to risk a possible three-minute romp. I wasn't a desperate twenty-year-old, so I wasn't at the point of no return to let him put it in. When he didn't insist on it, I was convinced he wouldn't be able to stand at attention for long.

"Well, then, can I taste you?" he pleaded, planting soft damp kisses behind my ears. He wanted to go south and serve himself a dish of me.

"No, I don't really like *that* that much," I said lying, knowing that once he did the pleasure of it would dictate my coming back for more and I did not want to be attached like that to him, though he was crazy about me. I liked my freedom of not having to answer to anyone or feeling the potential of being emotionally tethered to Luke. Relationships required commitment and responsibility and I just wasn't having it at that point of my life! I felt guilt and power surge through me like electrical power in a storm.

We continued kissing and I felt like wet clay in his hands. The Hugo Boss was whopping me into submission.

"Can I taste you?" he pleaded again, in a voice deep and husky with desire.

"Okay. But only for a little while," I said, allowing him to believe everything we were doing was his idea.

My silk top and lace bra were already off; Luke carefully ran his graceful fingers up my thighs and pulled off my black rayon skirt. I don't know what made me tremble more—my religious convictions (jettisoned like my clothes on the floor) or Luke's smooth moves.

I lay back as his tongue engraved wet alphabets on my stomach, beginning with my navel and working its way down my shaking thighs. I felt like I was in a wind tunnel. He gently parted my thighs and dived his face deeply into my genitalia. His thick tongue was stiff as he was licking and sucking gently on my labia. I could barely breathe. I wanted to cry out, but I wouldn't because I didn't want him to know how good he was making me feel. I lay there trembling under his tongue like a naked person locked out of her house during a blizzard.

When he found my clitoris, his mouth became a low speed motor and he suckled me as if I were a treat he'd never taste again. He was on a mission to bring me to an ecstasy I hadn't experienced in years. He sounded like a hungry hound feasting on a free kill. I began moving to the rhythm of his lips and tongue, and soon found myself climaxing. It happened so fast and furious, I was like a cocaine rat during a lab experiment. I went back for more and more until my clitoris was throbbing and exhausted from multiple climaxes. Luke was none the wiser. I had utterly enjoyed myself. He didn't even ask me to do him. It was as if he was satisfied for bringing me so much pleasure. I was too spent. This sealed things in his mind. He was a man in love and now he was messing with my schedule.

I liked Luke a lot, but not enough to get tangled into a long-term relationship. Yet, I found myself tipping over to his place to get satisfied at least once a week. He didn't care what I didn't do for him. My kissing him was enough. He told me he'd never been kissed like that. He was only too happy for me to serve him a meal of myself. He ate greedily until I stopped going to see him—I was becoming too attached. I ended us as abruptly as we had begun. Even now if I call him, he is too happy to pick up where we left off.

Ana Garza G'z

Jalapeño Jam

The peppers are perfect for stroking,
long, hard, smooth, the right fit
for the hand that slides over
them in the produce bin and curls
under their hanging fullnesses
between the stiff limbs of the capsicum
bush in the vegetable garden. How tempting

for the mouth that wants to close around and suck
the tip even as the knife breaks
the skin and the fingers burn
in lines to the palm where the seeds spill—
again—

even as the blender jar fills, turning
the cider vinegar jewel green, even as the boiling,
the sugar, the more cider vinegar, Pectin,
more Pectin, more....

And there it is, thick
and gemlike for crackers over a bed
of creamed cheese, quivering
to be consumed, to be rolled
between the tongue and the palate, to be held

for savoring. There it draws the saliva, engorging
the lips; tingling the roof of the mouth,
the gums, the swelling places inside
the cheeks; blunting the tactile for extreme
sensation, only to peak

in the absence of heat,
just sugar: cool
coupling without desire.

PERIE LONGO

THE WIDOW BECOMES UNDONE

At the fundraiser, she thought she should get something
out of IT, as the 17th century English used to say,
a stranger's eyes pure magnet as he smiled at her,
one of those smiles that makes your stomach dive.

She stood balanced on the tall, round table
created solely for drinking wine and nibbling
provocative hors d'oeuvres of bruschetta
topped with chickpeas and oysters. A violinist
and harpist were planted between the bougainvillea
and orange trees to ease release of money.
Have you bid? he asked, his arm
gesturing at the art mounted on easels,
suddenly around her waist. Tipping toward him,
not minding the pressure, she lied
 nothing interested her. It had been a long time
since the last "one" with bad back
and allergy to her cat.

Maybe it was the wine. Definitely the wine,
Pinot Grigio grown high in the Alps,
the bar tender winked. Romeo pointed to the gift baskets.
Take a look at those.
She wove over to the table, signed up for the "Night on the Town,"
a one night stay for two at a romantic hotel.

He (in her ear): *If you win, you have to take me.*
She: I never win anything.
He: *Tonight might be your night.*

Suddenly she heard her name called.
The prize was hers.
I am yours, he said and kissed her in front of everyone.
She felt IT coming, the blush the same color
as the resilient sun plummeting,
the flush that rose from some asleep place
and when she noticed all eyes on them, applauding,
she pulled away, *I don't even know him.*

Everyone laughed and turned back
to biting pickled asparagus tips
as if this were nothing unusual, leaving her,
                 no Juliet, with—alas, too young Romeo.

POMEGRANATE

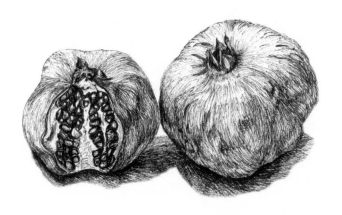

(tasting)

SUSAN LANDGRAF

SEVEN WOMEN AT THE TABLE

A WINDSTORM SHAKES the rafters, cedars and cattails in the pond outside the house. As we eat stuffed peppers and mixed greens, potatoes, the talk turns to vibrators—some simple as a penis-shaped head, circumcised plastic you can clean yourself, and others with two curves that with a little manipulation turn into a circle. One of us uses the simple kind. Another a device for extra stimulation during intercourse, which surprises one of us who can't imagine bringing up such a subject with her husband.

We do bring up the Republican presidential frontrunner, who says his is plenty enough to do the job, and we all agree there's been sex in the Oval Office but...on to the different shapes and costs of vibrators and whether to use lace or bare flesh for pre-play, one of us saying she used all of the above in her life long ago. Maybe, she says, the new ones will do more, and she'll think about it but doesn't want to go inside a dim, bulb-lit sex shop. One of us says you can find brightly lit shops with people who answer all your questions, just like shopping at AT&T for a phone. Speaking of which, you can activate some vibrators with your phone, and several of us slurp in our breath saying, *Really? What can't you do with your phone?* And laugh.

Imagine what they're thinking, the ones who track our every move, one of us says, and we don't laugh. Back and forth, our mouths full of stuffed peppers, mashed potatoes, wine, the presidential election, the fact that green peppers are unripe, red the ripest, yellow between, and the colors of vibrators, how women at a certain age don't talk about sex, one of us saying she'd been surprised years ago to learn intercourse meant both an exchange of thoughts and feelings as well as the sexual contact of genitalia, of anal and oral sex.

After a moment, one us quips *a pepper is a pepper is...but it isn't* another of us says and we fluctuate back and forth, the ones urging the others of us to discover what we've been missing, discuss the touch of flesh compared to plastic and the many meanings of communion but how the flesh betrays us—the walls of our vaginas thinning, for instance, just like our pubic hair when we get older, how sexual intercourse hurts unless you lubricate, the young ones among us open-mouthed in disbelief, one of us saying *no one's ever told me my vagina walls will thin*, so we go into creams, prescriptions, exercise.

Then we go on to the white cake with apricot filling. We drink wine while the wind rages, trees shed their branches or fall.

It is the night before the Ides of March, the presidential primary elections, and we all know where this is going, the Republican presidential candidates talking walls, guns, and one claiming he has compassion and answers. So we go back to vibrators and writing, seven women sitting at table, communing about how we'll return to our day jobs of giving voice in a world where we still have a choice about who we open to, who we let in, and how.

MARYAM ALA AMJADI

A TRUE TRIANGLE

Translated from Rira Abbasi's Farsi poem

Perhaps it is mistakenly simple
The water that is spilled
cannot be gathered into one drop
It is mistakenly simple
This is me, a true triangle
standing between some pointless floating words
It walks in me this triangle
It walks inside my loins
For years something yearns to make me crumble,
make me spill
It was love
It was the frothy fuming years of forty
It's still the same today,
but my neighbour says:
Triangles die fast, they die fast
I have no desire in death
Every Friday
Every month
Every year
and my downfall under that one point of the triangle...
I am upright and still erect under the points of this trinity,
but the neighbour falls in the footpath of my power,
so that I may fall
I am spilled from three words:
Girl
        Woman
Mother

and I still tremble between the fish of my thighs
What tradition of the neighbour should I follow that I may not fall?
Should I turn back and remain Maryam?

God

                Son
The Spirit of God

God is a full time boy
and only one of them becomes holy,
destiny or decided,
there is no sign of any triangle
I don't know, was my grandmother a full time Maryam?
Let this triangle, let everything become non-functional
even though the spirit hangs heady from my head
and the points of trinity are many
I become a grandmother and I still wander
Perhaps it is mistakenly simple,
but I will remind them, I will teach them
the water that is spilled
turns into my shape.

In Iran's popular culture, "Friday Night"—in reality, Thursday night, the night before Friday—is humorously regarded as the recommended time for copulation. The notion seems to have stemmed from practical religious treatises that mark auspicious days and timings for specific activities, including sex; "Maryam," here, equates to Virgin Mary.

DIANE RAPTOSH

VIEWS FROM A FORMER
CONTORTIONIST

She missed looking at mountains and seeing men in them, tens of
them maybe—rows of rough-hewn torsos waiting for her to finally
knuckle down. She wanted still to feel the need to mount them, one at
a time, to lay to, to undo their detachment, to back-stride every set of
jags on the Cascades, to hasp onto the furthest peaks of the Brabazon
Range and fall to work, one quick pump of every other point on the
Carpathians, whip hand not hanging on to anything. She missed the
need to think she had to do something swashy or wry with her tongue
on the west tip of the Rockies—bent up and scarp-faced, to lick out
the fusty, unseen rucks of so many folding contortionists, or, to do
something more rose-hued, like bleed all over the pointiest part of Los
Cuernos del Paine in southern Chile or ease slowly down the nose of
each face in the Presidential Range. She yearned to long again for the
mass of the great great Grampians in Oceania lying in wait beneath
her, for the Slovene Karavanke chain to openly slake her liquid need.
Not to mention effects of thinking of the Montes Recti and Mons
Hansteen—mountains on the moon—ready for just such scenes to
come to fruition. Nor to mention Cuba's Sierra Maestra: She'd always
wanted to hover just over that mother-idea.

Lisa del Rosso

The Man from Kentucky

He walked me to my mother's condo, but I wanted to say goodbye in the parking lot, rather than in front of her door. I was fifty, after all, not fifteen.

It was the end of my spring break in March 2016, and I had not planned on seeing him again, thinking that our differences were insurmountable. We had three great dates, but that last walk on the beach, with humidity rising and grey storm clouds rolling in on the Gulf, I thought that a number of things I tried to talk about, namely my book and agents and publishers, he either ignored, or did not or could not respond. I could not tell which. If this sounds like I am a snob, you are right: I am a snob, and not only because I am a professor at NYU and have lived in London and New York City for a combination of thirty-two years.

So, in the parking lot and eager to get rid of him, I quickly stuck my hand out (those three great dates were also chaste) to say goodbye.

Easy.

Except, he did not respond in kind. Instead, he took my hand, kissed it and said very slowly, in that pronounced Southern accent,

"Lisa, all I want to do is to make love to you and I really DIG YOU."
When he said, "dig you" he made a bird-like motion with his hands
and pointed at me. Then he turned and walked away.

I have no idea how long I stood there. Could have been a minute,
could have been two. I know I can draw the back view of his broad
shoulders in the gray T-shirt he was wearing, along with the black
shorts and black and grey sneakers until he was in the distance,
then no longer visible. He didn't look back, but had he turned and
glanced over his shoulder, he might have wondered why I looked as
if I had just been hit by a bus.

No man had ever said that to me.

Let me rephrase: no man has ever said that to me and been dead
serious about what he was saying.

This man was *serious*. But he lives in Florida. I live in New York
City. And we are complete opposites.

But when he said, "Lisa, all I want to do is to make love to you
and I really DIG YOU," my response was entirely physical. I felt
something give in my heart and something give in my shorts at the
same time.

Uh-oh.

From that moment, I knew that whatever it was that I felt, it
was unfinished. That day, I got on the plane back to NYC and he
began texting me.

Every single morning.

At first, I thought it was delightful, then unusual, then nuts,
then unsustainable, and then I so looked forward to them that one
day when he was late, I missed them terribly.

In the age of technology, I would call this Wooing Via Text
(WVT).

Kentucky, my nickname for him, had told me his fiftieth
birthday was May 17. My school term ended on May 9, and wouldn't
you know, I have summers off. So I casually mentioned I had some
time off and if he could get free for a day or two, maybe I could
come down and see him for his birthday. We looked at some dates.
Then I got this text: "I think so highly of you I rearranged my whole

vacation [normally a week in August] so I could spend time with you."

Did I mention that I have made all of the major decisions in my life, for better or worse, in under three seconds?

1. Moving to London
2. Moving to New York City
3. Becoming a teacher.
4. Booking my flight.

He also asked his boss of twenty-one years to borrow a small efficiency apartment on the beach, only for me, not for him, and this was granted.

My mother of seventy-three has learned how to text. This newly acquired skill is now the bane of my life. After all this transpired with Kentucky, we engaged in the following annotated text conversation:

Tuesday, March 22

Mom: Don't you think you are moving a little fast with a man you hardly know?

Me: I have two months to get to know him via text and phone. I can't get to know him in person unless I spend some time there or he spends some time here. I am not staying with him (he, like me, has a roommate). So, if after a week, we hate each other, or our worlds are too different, then at least I will know. And he will, too. If I don't at least try, I'll never know: nothing lost, nothing gained.

Tuesday, March 29th

Me: Kentucky called a little while ago and I actually feel a whole lot better now. He arranged the rental with his boss and it is free: he has the key and is checking the place out tomorrow. If it's awful, he'll arrange something else. I am not used to a man saying, "I'll take care of it" and actually taking care of it. I am used to the opposite, and Yash [my ex-husband] used to do it all the time—say he'd do something then not do it. Drove me crazy. And as you know, I took care of everything of this nature—trips, accommodation, transport, tickets—because if I didn't, no one would. The fact is, I have done everything for myself for such a long time and am so fiercely independent, I no longer trust any man to do anything. But surprisingly, Kentucky has taken care of it, and, like, wow. I think I'm in shock.

Mom: Good for him. I hope you have a lot in common with him. I'm sure he's a nice guy, but I wonder if he has your love of books, plays and the arts to keep you interested. You are a very smart woman!

Me: Probably not. But I had all that in common with Yash and the marriage didn't work. You also are a very smart woman, and you and Steve [my stepfather] are very different. The marriage works. Maybe opposites attract? I don't know. As I said, the dates were good dates, which is not something I am used to. I am used to passive men or liars or narcissists. Maybe having everything in common is not necessary. I know I'd rather be with someone honest, opinionated, who knows who they are and does what they say they are going to do. And also is not afraid of life, of new possibilities. And not afraid of being a man.

Mom (after a pause): Good point.

Earlier that month I had gone down to visit my mother and stepfather in Venice, Florida, as I have for the past fifteen years. Every year, I go to Bresler's Ice Cream shop to buy iced coffee, which is both delicious and giant-sized, roughly sixteen ounces for two dollars (unheard of in New York City). The shop is airy and white with flamingo-pink wrought-iron seats; it smells yummy, because they make their own cones on the premises, and the menfolk behind the counter are always pleasant, chatty, complimentary, and sometimes flirtatious. I walk in feeling okay and leave with the over-inflated ego of a super model—that's how skillfully these men wield their flattery. Kentucky, the manager, is usually the one who waits on me.

We have talked and flirted, and talked and flirted. For years. And for years, while also noticing the absence of a wedding ring, I have wondered why the man never asked me out for a drink, a meal, or even an ice cream cone. One year, he had a cross around his neck, and so I thought he was likely a deeply religious person who was looking for another deeply religious person, which I am not. Or, he was celibate, like a priest, which I am not. A year later, no cross. So I remained puzzled, yet pleased when he told me I was beautiful, and kept leaving the shop with only my giant-sized coffee.

In March 2016, I went down for my annual visit. And as usual, on the first day, I went to Bresler's for an iced coffee. Behind the counter was a server I had seen the year before: Jimmy, a striking man of sixty-nine with white hair, a white goatee, bright blue eyes and a Southern accent. He went in immediately:

"You need to be coming here every day. Please do."

"You need to move down here; we need you down here."

"If I were thirty-five years younger, I'd chase you all over the state of Florida."

"You're just beautiful."

Kentucky, meanwhile, ran around getting my coffee, nodding in agreement with everything Jimmy said. When he handed it to me, he said, "You're beautiful."

I left with my coffee.

Halfway through my visit, on a Wednesday, during a Bresler's stop, Jimmy, while appraising me from top to bottom, said, "Miss Lisa? I'm going to ask you something that I shouldn't ask but I'm going to ask anyway."

I said, "Okay."

He said, "I've noticed you wear no wedding ring on your left hand."

I said, "Right."

He said, "You're not married?"

I said, "No, I'm not.

He fairly shouted, "WHAT IS WRONG WITH THE MEN IN NEW YORK CITY?"

I laughed. Then I said, "Well, the men in New York City by and large want twenty-one-year-olds, and that's not me, and I don't care!"

He said, "They must be out of their minds. If I were a younger man...."

By that time, I had gotten to the register, and Jimmy asked if I had children. I said I was divorced with no children. Kentucky, who had been silent and, I hoped, listening to all of this, stuck out his hand as if to shake mine and said, "Divorced, no children, no baggage!"

I laughed again, shook his hand and said, "Me, too!"

He said, "You come down here every year, right?"

I said yes.

He said, "We should get together and go out."

I said, "That would be great."

Thursday night, I met him for dinner, which happened to be St. Patrick's Day, so the city was nuts. We went to one place and the noise level was apparent from the sidewalk; once in, I asked the hostess, "How loud is it out there?" She said it was pretty loud, and it would take ten minutes for a table.

"Let's go," I said.

As we crossed the street to go to his first choice, he said, "Lisa, man, you've really got it together."

I said, "What makes you say that?"

He said, "Most women don't."

The date was great, because it was a proper date. Much later, when we said goodbye, I kissed him, but he was smiling, so no reciprocal kiss.

I went in. I paced the guest bedroom. No kiss bothered me. So I texted him.

Friday night, I met him for a drink, then a walk, and we wound up sitting on a bench by the sea under the moonlight. We talked. And talked and talked. Kentucky went to U of Michigan on a basketball scholarship, and all was well till he blew out his knee. No more scholarship, so no more university. He went to college in Sarasota, but never finished. Later, I found out that even though he has no degree *and I have three*, as a manager he makes far and away more money than I do. This is the way it is in America.

It was a beautiful night. We were on the bench together for perhaps an hour, perhaps more. And he still didn't kiss me.

Walking back to the car, he kept talking until I said, "Shut up and kiss me."

Yay!

He unlocked the ice cream shop and ate Key Lime Pie frozen yogurt behind the counter (in addition to the cones, they also make all their own ice cream, topping, etc., on the premises). He said something about being nervous the night before, or jittery, or intimidated, which made me laugh, so I kissed him again, which was nice. And I liked his arm around my waist.

When we said goodnight, no kiss.

WTF?

Saturday, the day I was leaving, Kentucky asked if he could see me for a walk or breakfast or both, so we went to the beach and walked.

On days that involve me getting on a plane, I am irritable, anxious and distracted. I love arriving, but hate traveling. I hate packing. I hate airports. I hate everything traveling involves.

So on the beach with those billowing storm clouds in the distance, impatient that Kentucky didn't get every reference or detail I threw at him, I decided I wouldn't keep in touch and instead remain friendly. I'd stop by for iced coffee when I was in town. But I didn't think he was the man for me.

Until we said goodbye.

Tanya Ko Hong

Denied

After fifty, I should want nothing
Your kiss, your touch, your embrace
not even the smile that says
I know you, Wife,
I should not want to speak
my mouth should be a stone
on this pillow beside you

But my mouth is soft
and open with longing
hungry to taste you
betraying my need.

I want you to love me
under the moonlight
on top of a mountain
that looks over lakes
over borderlines
not just to please you
but to please me
to know my body well
the body I didn't know
how to love

Even stones yearn
flowers growing between them
glowing the deep tree roots
breaking apart with life
sweetness pushing through like song.

ROBERTA FEINS

THE CONFINED NATURE OF BODILY SENSATION

Had I been born crested and not cloven my lords,
you would not have treated me thus.

~

Spare the rib, and then where's Eve?

~

With proper care, your dryer
should give you years of service.
Just give her a good swift kick.

~

Madam Secretary, I'd like to add
my lust to the agenda.

~

If a woman cries in the Ladies Room,
what's the point? He's not going to know.

~

Among mysterious pipes and gears
I would someday move easily: switches, kisses.

~

Cynical, ashamed, unchaste and odd,
I had to tell bawdy stories to all his friends.

~

When you kissed me, I snapped like the flag.

~

Always the intro scene with the wagon and chorus.

~

Pushing through a crowd of boys,
a hand on my breast, laughter.

~

You always pretended the past was lovely
But what shaped your life were shadows.

Rita Bullinger

Talk Juicy: Love and Lust at Sixty-plus

In 2014, at the age of sixty-four, an unexpected event changed my life. I'd bought a house that April, the sycamores on my front lawn reminders of my Midwestern childhood, and in late summer a man I'd wanted to know better—as in way better—reappeared. We'd met a year earlier at a sustainability course in north Oakland, offered by an adjunct professor we both knew. I was drawn to him like a magnet; I found myself, regressed schoolgirl, just wanting to sit next to him. Even after I found out he was married.

2013 had been a year of other changes as well: I'd excavated myself from the celibate dungeon of a marriage gone terribly awry (that ended in divorce, of course); I'd pushed away the webs of alcohol addiction; I'd joined a recovery therapy group; and my work was going well. When Isis, my daughter's cairn terrier, and I moved into my first solely purchased home (without the bank roll of a spouse), I was randy for companionship. I flirted awkwardly with the handy man, almost had sex with the young African-American Comcast guy, and landed in a sort-of relationship with a man who is now my friend—what our relationship should have been from the start minus my desperate sex yearnings.

I remember well Rhett's first foray into my life as an unmarried man. Standing outside on the lawn of a lovely little church in Kensington, where I was talking to a twelve-step friend and probably smoking a cigarette, living what I think of as my "hallway" life—stuck between my false self and my True Self—Rhett texted me. I looked down to see his name on my iPhone screen. I squealed a girly shout of pure delight. Never in a hundred reincarnations did I expect to hear from this man.

I felt exonerated somehow that I hadn't imagined his attraction to me. Later, he told me he knew I was "trouble." He told me he had begun to mentally undress me when he overheard me say I loved the freedom of walking around my house naked.

The text asked if I wanted to have brunch; he told me later that his wife was divorcing him and he was expanding his "friend group"—for thirty years his life had revolved around his wife and kids. I couldn't do brunch, but suggested dinner in the next week. Across the table at an outdoor café on Telegraph Avenue, I looked at this tall, handsome man and felt a vague indifference born of fear. Why, I wondered, would I want to have any sort of relationship with a man who had just been dumped by his wife, to whom he still wanted to be married?

That attraction I'd felt for him throughout the course and even after when I'd invited him to join a guerrilla theatre group I was forming seemed to have fizzled. Later, at my house over tea and conversation, I convinced myself I wasn't in the least attracted to him. But Rhett was relentless. He invited me to listen to a lecture series he was giving in a neighboring city and we drove together and then ate dinner afterward. Our relationship grew.

At the time, I'd been reading Caroline and Charles Muir's classic book on tantra, an ancient sexual practice in which couples focus on breathing, chakra consciousness, and not coming to orgasm but instead hoarding orgasmic energy to stay sexy and connected. I'd also read a book by Jewish Rabbi Shmuley Boteach titled *Kosher Sutra* (an international bestseller) and had been captivated by his notion of the female as a goddess of pleasure and the source of divine energy. I'd loved reading about men needing to honor women's sensual, passionate, and intuitive guidance during love-making, and this notion that lust—especially in marriage—is absolutely mandatory for any long-lasting relationship to stay juicy. No wonder I'd divorced.

I soon recommended both books to Rhett and he immediately ordered them on his Kindle. He later said his first impression about me had been proven true—that I was a woman who enjoyed sex. Maybe, but I knew I couldn't be in a relationship with Rhett the way I'd been in relationships in the past.

Over the course of a year, Rhett and I grew closer with several fits and starts along the way. We began a sexual relationship built on friendship and mutual trust, he bought a house near mine, and we began to figure out how to remain juicy.

So far so good.

At this writing we've been together for two years. Here's what's working for us:

1. We don't live together;

2. We have separate bank accounts, mortgages, friends, interests, activities, and opinions (we also have friends in common);

3. We work on our relationship via a process called Imago Dialogue;

4. We are both semi-retired;

5. We share many interests such as eco-sustainability, progressive politics, commitment to neighborhood arts and small business start-ups, and entertaining;

6. We are in a committed, monogamous relationship;

7. Should we break up, we want to remain life-long friends (really!).

Both Rhett and I have been in marriages where sex became a solitary affair—masturbating in the shower, cumming alone with a vibrator, pretending to be asleep—and have felt that lonely despair of wanting connection but not getting it, sometimes for years.

Yes, our relationship is relatively new and that may be why our sex life is so juicy. Still, we both believe if we continue to stay connected, we will remain passionate and eager in bed. We're also aware that not living together helps. As a friend of Rhett's noted, "You and Rita, unlike most of us, aren't focused on how to get away from each other; instead you guys want to know 'when can we get together again?'"

Rhett and I both get to say when we want to be together and for how long. And it works miraculously, for, after all, we aren't raising children together, he sleeps better separately, I like my writer's solitude, we live only six doors away so if I need him or he needs me getting together is easy, and neither of us requires the other's financial help.

Bottom line: Rhett and I are both sensual people. We engage in a practice called "Fuck First" or FF (from an article in The Huffington Post: the idea being FF before wine and dinner because afterward you're too tired and full) and which we've adapted to include "Skin Time" or ST. Skin Time means we want to just touch without sex. ST helps eliminate any fear or guilt that we won't be able to perform to the expectations of our partner. We use these acronyms in our texts asking for "FF and dinner?" or "ST b4 Berkeley Rep?"

We genuinely love to feel the silk of our skin beneath the palpable hunger of our fingers and our lips. We enjoy being touched and touching. We make dates to do so. And, wondrously and genuinely, I have taken a hankering to oral sex. Being an eager devotee of the olfactory sense, I love the smell of his genitals and the feel of his cock and balls in my mouth. His response is such a turn-on! I've done quite a bit of experimenting with Rhett and believe that the way to a man's heart is through his appetite to be sucked and sucked well. (Note: the woman has to genuinely love cock sucking. This one can't be faked.)

But here's the thing: the juicy sex we are having now probably doesn't have much to do with pheromones, his delight in my breasts, or the fact that I "sit geisha" beside him cradling his genitals as he fondles me. What makes sex juicy for us is the quality of our conversations. That's right. Communication coupled with oral sex, I'm convinced, is what makes sex at sixty-six the best sex of our lives.

Arousal for both of us begins and ends with our commitment to letting each other be different, be ourselves, and speak our truth. We engage in something called "Imago dialogue," a process a psychotherapist named Harville Hendrix first outlined in a popular book titled, *Getting the Love You Want*. Briefly, it works like this: Rita brings up a topic or concern, states as clearly as she can what it is. Rita and Rhett make time as soon as possible to sit and dialogue. Rita, who brought up the topic, talks first, and Rhett, after centering in his safe world where he has been invited to walk across a bridge to Rita's world, and is a guest in her world, listens and mirrors.

Mirroring means Rhett states what Rita has said as succinctly as possible, using exact words from her share—that is, no interpretation wanted or needed. When Rita has finished speaking and Rhett has mirrored along the way, Rhett asks, "Is there more?" Then, if there is more, Rhett continues to listen and mirror. Finally, Rhett summarizes what he heard, validates that Rita's world view makes sense (even if he doesn't *agree* with it), and offers empathy. And then the roles switch, and Rita listens to Rhett: mirrors, validates, and empathizes.

What woman does not get juicy when her partner asks her, "Is there more?" My God, thank you, Jesus! Is there *more?* Yes, there's always more—women have so much more to say, because women want, more than anything, to simply be listened to, understood, and still wanted and desired. At least this woman does. Once that happens outside the bedroom, what happens inside the bedroom makes those silly Viagra ads appear as sterile and banal as they are.

What typically occurs after Rhett and I dialogue is an opening of vulnerability, trust, and what we call juice. Rhett and I are already keenly attracted to each other physically and sexually, emotionally and intellectually—so that foundation exists and has from the beginning. After dialogue, our juicy feelings seem super-powered.

I feel even more known, rather than shut off, shut up, or merely tolerated—common feelings from past relationships. Often, Rhett and I embrace and kiss passionately after a dialogue, then head to the bedroom.

Once in bed, emotionally open, we are eager to appreciate each other's aging bodies, both overweight and bountiful, sensual and sweet. Rhett appreciates my breasts and pussy with his words (always a turn-on), his mouth and tongue, and his hands. I appreciate his butt and chest, his cock and balls in similar ways. We both appreciate each other's eyes, hair, legs, whatever it is we love about the other—and say so out loud.

Again, we communicate with our words and I think this is key to our getting-better-every-day sex life. We talk. We also act. Move. Play. Experiment. Do. Breathe. Laugh. Practice. Ask. The art of asking is crucial. I cannot read Rhett's mind and he can't read mine. While it may be difficult, embarrassing, silly, or whatever, asking is essential to juicy lovemaking.

Another crucial talking point, often unspoken by women, is penis size. But this topic has been a stab of contention and comparison for men their entire lives. For this reason, I think it's really important to admire your partner's package often. Rhett's penis is perfect and I tell him so frequently. But, since both my belly and Rhett's need trimming down, penetration sometimes isn't easy to accomplish. We tried it early in our relationship and both separated in a heap of laughter and acceptance. Not being fucked or fucking in the traditional sense is a non-issue for us. I know Rhett likes me to pay attention to his cock from the get-go. I want more of a lead-up. But, sometimes, I want his long, generous fingers to fuck me hard right away since I am wet and ache for penetration. Without hesitation, Rhett obliges.

Rhett is a sensuous and generous lover. He pays attention to what I want by listening to my breathing, my words, and my moans. Kissing well is central to our pleasure. Rhett says when he kisses my lips it's "like coming home." Rhett is available to me at every phase of our lovemaking, and since I clear up any feelings I might have of being manipulated, controlled, any feelings of anger, disrespect, shame, self-doubt, or fear—and he does the same with his list, which usually centers around my victim stuff, perceived invasiveness, or his need for autonomy and privacy, we don't usually bring into the bedroom those emotional lead-weights that burden most couples from natural feelings of spontaneity, lust, and friendship.

One of my favorite fantasies is that I'm seventeen and he's seventeen and we are making love as teenagers with all the curiosity and candor we naturally had then (even if we didn't have the loving and generous partners we are for each other now). We also don't harbor a need to cum. Orgasms aren't that urgent for us. We are in it for the pleasure in the moment and if we orgasm, we do, and if we don't, no biggie. It's arousal and lust that gets us juicy and where, as in tantric sex, holding back from cumming is a whole lot sexier.

This is the luxury—and freedom—of loving in these sixty-plus years. I'm keenly aware of my own desire to *really* love this beautiful man who entered my life and has changed me, entirely, for the better. It's easy to ask myself: What does he like? How would he enjoy this? When I open up more, how does it affect his pleasure? If intimacy means truly listening to another, that leads to daring to ask: Does this feel good? What do you want now? How about this? And, absolutely essential, it means listening to one's own desires in the physical moment-to-moment act of sexual love. Breathe in. Breathe out.

For Rhett and me, it feels good to enjoy oral sex, to fondle and touch, but refrain from cumming. We feel lusty a good amount of the time. We kiss passionately often and as our relationship lengthens we affirm our desire to continue to remain juicy and available, as well as open to new positions, areas of eroticism yet unexplored (like anal sex), and our changing appetites and desires. Surprises are fun, too—like the time Rhett opened the door completely naked. My turn next!

MARIANNE PEEL

IT WOULDN'T BE MAKE BELIEVE IF YOU BELIEVED IN ME

For Blanche Dubois

You want me to give you lemon coke with ice chips
To soothe you in your jagged places
A hot drawn bath
In the throbbing heat
Of the French Quarter.

But I have wanted
to bathe with you in lavender water
Adorned with water lilies
Your feather boa transformed into ringlets of water pearls
Caressing your neck your shoulders
The lattice lace of your hair
Gathered around a musical mouth
That hums only love songs.

I have wanted
To be moored with you in this harbor,
The stranger you depend on
For kindness.
We will banish all naked light bulbs,
Dressing them in Chinese lanterns from the five and dime.
At midnight we will read love letters
From your long ago lover
Remembering the New Orleans jazz trumpet
How it lured you to the dance floor
How you kicked off your heels
How your hips couldn't help but sway and swish

How the smoke curled in and out of your eyes.

I have wanted
Letters from that lover
In our water-puckered hands
Just reading and remembering.
Not make-believe.
Knowing we tell what ought to be truth.

Missy Michaels

Turned On

I HAD MY FIRST real orgasm at fifty-one.

Until only very recently, I had not had sex in more than three years. Once upon a time, my partner of more than twenty years and I had sex fairly regularly. And, for the record, he was one of the more attentive lovers I had been with, and I will be honest and say that there had been more than I can count. While I was never wildly attracted to him, I was attracted to the fact that he desired me.

At the age of thirty, I experienced my first orgasm with him, which, on reflection, was probably closer to a vaginal sneeze than a full-blown orgasm, but I was, for the most part, pretty happy with that given that most of my prior sexual encounters involved minimal foreplay and speedy, and mostly deeply unsatisfying, intercourse.

After a traumatic and lengthy delivery with our first son, our sex life resumed but with reduced gusto until we hit an impasse as to whether or not we would, should or could have a second child. I had wrongly assumed that of course we would; he was not so sure. We stopped talking about it, and even though we continued to have sex, it was always with a condom until one fateful night when at the age of forty-two, after just one unprotected fuck, I got pregnant. If

I had to mark a point on a map as to when our lives changed, it was probably then.

When my son turned four he was diagnosed with autism. I think it's fair to say that sexual desire and Autism Spectrum Disorders are not the greatest bedfellows, and so my libido was fast disappearing as my anxiety about the future increased. They were heartbreaking months. I had my hands full to overflowing trying to unravel the complexity of the diagnosis, and what his challenges, and therefore what our challenges, might be. As if this wasn't hard enough, this chapter coincided with the sinking realization that my partner (Mr. A) was not stepping up to the plate. I felt as though I was traveling this path alone. Until that point in our relationship, I had been pretty patient with his annoying quirks and general inflexibility, but the moment he decided to have himself assessed for Asperger's tipped me over the edge. I had no patience or energy left in my depleted tank for this new and ultimately not very helpful revelation.

This was another red flag on the map of our deteriorating journey. It was only a couple of years ago that it occurred to me not only had I not had sex for more than two years, I had forgotten that at one time I quite liked sex. While I never thought too deeply about my sexuality, I took it as normal that men found me sexually attractive. What was more worrying was this lack of sex drive did not concern me. I told myself that I'd become celibate, and felt almost virtuous. When my friend suggested it might be a good time to buy a vibrator, I felt this was almost scandalous, but furtively ordered one online. While it was moderately pleasurable, akin to those vaginal sneezes I used to experience, I got quickly bored; finding I was more interested in checking Facebook.

Around this time, that same friend told me about a practice called OM (orgasmic meditation). Essentially, it is a meditative practice that involves "a stroker" giving absolute focus to a woman's clitoris. The theory behind it is that women are so hard-wired to be caretakers that many of us have shut down our sexuality. In order for us to feel nourished and alive, we need oxytocin, the love hormone that fires us up sexually and creatively. The idea is being in a state of orgasm is essential to a woman's sense of self. On a practical level, the practice involves the woman removing the bottom half of her clothing and allowing a man to stroke her clitoris or "pussy" for fifteen minutes. I was intrigued and slightly appalled, but shelved it for another time.

In April 2015, I turned fifty. Instead of having a party, I decided to have a women's ritual to mark this new phase of my life. It was an incredible, life-affirming experience, surrounded by amazing women who love me, and were there to remind me of my value and worth. I created a slide show for the occasion, and among the many childhood photos I found pictures of old boyfriends, most significantly, my dreadlocked black lover (Mr. V) from two decades ago when I lived in New York. I felt turned on just looking at the photos. I wondered what it would be like to be with him after all these years. While we had been in some contact on social media over the years, I never really considered that I might see him again.

In the face of massive opposition from Mr. A, I decided, as a birthday present to myself, that I would attend a writing workshop with my all-time favorite writer on a Greek island. Leaving my family for the first time, I felt like an escapee from my domestic prison. I had arrived in paradise.

I had a vague thought that since I was on this grand adventure, maybe I could make contact with Mr. V, and see if he was up for a Greek island fling. Back in Australia, all my friends insisted I watch "Shirley Valentine"—which I have to say was a rather depressing film. But the main character does walk away from her domestic drudgery, have a bit of sexy fun in the sun, and lives happily ever after.

I never did contact Mr. V, but ended up happily surrounded by a posse of fabulous women, many of whom were lesbians. I was so buzzed by this adventure I entertained the idea that maybe this fantasy fling could swing either way. However, despite the best intentions of my new pals in Patmos, I remained a Patmos virgin.

My girth had increased significantly in recent years, and while I tried not to focus on that, my body image was not at an all time high. I had refused to subscribe to the idea that a woman over a certain age, becomes invisible, yet, I felt as though I was slipping into that sexless quicksand of invisibility.

I was starting to mourn the person who used to attract men like bees to honey.

I returned from this adventure with renewed zeal that somehow I needed to fight for this spark as though my life depended on it. Which it did.

Meanwhile, back on the home front, my family was struggling to recognize me. I was always the mother who would drive everyone everywhere, feed anyone anytime, and rarely said no to anyone. You could say that I was completely without boundaries. And here I was, waltzing off to Greece, putting myself first. Mr. A never recovered from this outrageous and deeply defiant act. So when, several months later, I announced that I was going to the U.S to do *another* writing workshop, he put his headphones on and pretended I had not said a word.

Meanwhile, my sexually adventurous buddy had taken to OM with gusto and was encouraging me to be brave and join the action. For the next few months, I became the resident OM expert to all my other pals. And even though I was not yet courageous enough to actually sign up, I was pretty curious.

The year rolled around, and I tentatively booked and paid my airfare to attend a writing workshop in Big Sur, knowing I was going to be held to emotional ransom for my decision, but also knowing it was taking a monumental step toward following my own desires.

As we touched down in San Francisco, I felt like I'd been plugged into a light socket, and an electrical current was recharging my body. I couldn't sleep. My usually robust appetite vanished and I once again found myself turned on by being so far from the duties of motherhood, and excited by the idea that I was in the U.S. after nearly two decades. After a year of Skype calls and emails I was back in the same room with some of my favorite people from my Greek adventure, and this too was quite overwhelming. I was turned on by everything and everyone.

I had sent Mr. V a message saying I would be coming to the West Coast, and asked if he wanted to catch up. He said "of course" and I left it at that. There had always been other women in the picture, and even though he told me he was not married, I had no reason to think anything would be any different twenty years on.

I deliberately left the last few days of my trip open, as I had originally planned to go to LA. As it happened, I had no reason to go there other than to see him, so when he contacted me, I was pretty direct. I knew if I saw him, there was no question we would sleep together. Over the phone he told me it might be complicated for me to stay with him as he had been in a twelve-year relationship with a very possessive and very married Iranian woman. I suggested that we forget about the liaison, but he made it clear he wanted to see me. After countless messages, we agreed he would drive to Monterey and meet at a hotel. I was incredibly nervous and excited. It was my first opportunity to have sex in a long time. I wondered if he would still find me attractive after nearly two decades, and more important, me, him.

He drove through the night arriving at 8 a.m. From the moment I saw him I knew the spark was still alive. He went down on me before we'd had a chance to stop and look at each other. While this was my fantasy come true, I was equally bewildered by the lack of intimacy in this act. I was incredibly turned on by this, by him, but it made me sad that he really couldn't look at me. I was seeing him through a new filter. Sure, I was like a hungry tiger, wanting to devour and be devoured, but I felt some disappointment. This was not going to be a quick and meaningless fuck, but neither was it going to be a deep and tender exchange.

What was I expecting?

We spent most of the weekend in our luxurious king-size bed, sometimes talking about our lives, but mostly fooling around, so I was surprised when this virile black man couldn't keep an erection. Quite truthfully, I was fine with all the other stuff, which I have always found preferable to feeling like a tire being pumped. I made a confession that I had never looked at porn, a fact that he felt compelled to rectify, and so we had fun, mixing that into the bedroom recipe. As there was some blood on the sheets, he asked me if I had my period. I laughed and said, "I hope so," as my periods have waxed and waned for some time. He looked confused, and when I said the word "menopause," he shook his head in disbelief, saying that I was too ripe to be at that stage of life. While it was flattering, it made me wonder if he had any real idea about middle age, mine or his own.

When he left to drive back to LA in the middle of the night I thought I was okay, but truthfully I felt like I had been cracked open. While I knew I was incredibly brave for allowing myself to be so vulnerable, I was also starting to realize this encounter would be both devastating and liberating.

I cried all the way home to Australia. I told him I felt as though an old wound had been re-opened, a notion I think he understood but preferred not to be drawn into.

As soon as I got home, I decided this would be the perfect time to experiment with this OM thing. I was going to need all the oxytocin I could get.

I knew I did not want to remain within the ranks of sexless middle-aged women who sublimate their desires with chocolate and pinot noir. I both wanted and needed to feel sexual.

I made some calls and, while I was not quite brave enough to sign up for the group training session, I booked two private sessions with the incredibly smart and wise-beyond-her-years OM coach. I expected to be more nervous than I was. More concerned if I needed to get a Brazilian, shave or go *au naturel* than I was about the prospect of a stranger stroking my pussy.

There I was, an OM virgin, lying on the floor, naked from the waist down, with a very kind and gentle man taking instruction from my OM coach about how to stroke me. I tried to relax and get in the zone, but found it hard to be turned on while lying on the floor in a strange room, with a timer and a woman I've just met coaching my "stroker" to "stay on top of the orgasm." I didn't feel especially orgasmic, but was proud of myself for having gone through with it.

I was not yet convinced this was for me. It reminded me more of a visit to the gynecologist than an erotic event.

For my follow-up session, I asked another man I had never met to attend. The first things I noticed were his piercing dark eyes, a striking, long, curly moustache, and unbridled sexual energy. Instantly, I felt the crackle of electricity. This time I wanted to experience two OMs as I was pretty sure that it might take some time to relax and "let go." During the second OM, Mr. Piercing Dark Eyes started to make a growling sound, and this time I felt pretty turned on.

Officially an OM graduate, I was invited into the strange alternate universe of OM. There are various Facebook threads where the protocol is to ask someone if they would like to OM, always being clear that they can say "yes" or "no," as can I. But being brave is the name of the game here, so I contacted Mr. Piercing Dark Eyes to ask if he would like to OM with me again. He said he would, and as fate or Freud would have it, my mother had just gone overseas, so we met at her apartment. We talked for a bit, and then we OM'd. Again, the first time was hard for me to let myself go, but when we finished, I cried. I had that feeling again of being cracked open, but this time it was not by anyone else, it was all mine. The second OM turned a corner. The phone rang and I could hear my mother on the answering machine, and I laughed at the absurdity of it all. Meanwhile my body was quivering with pleasure as I had my first real orgasm.

Having only been OM'ing for a few weeks, my body is tingling with sensations I have not experienced in years. I seriously wonder if I have crossed over to the "dark side." Now I fit in OM sessions before picking up my son from school, and have a smile on my face in spite of the challenges I face on the domestic front. At the age of fifty-one, I feel like the switch has at last been turned *on*.

LOIS MARIE HARROD

IN THE MUSEUM OF FUCKING

The lighting varies
from room to room—
sometimes so direct
you can see
the loons and seagulls
spread their seams,
sometimes so pitch
you feel your way
through spine
and prickle
to flaccid deep,
sometimes so dusk
you can taste
the moon's lozenge
as it slips down
to the wet bottom
of the sea
where creatures
you have just begun
to imagine
propagate
in steamy vents,
and everywhere
you breathe
the diaphanous
odors of musk
and mayhem,
and each exhibit
you pass says
please ~~do not~~ touch

but not here, here,
and you keep touching
here and here
and now here.

LORI WHITE

I CHOSE AN EASTERN KING

ORIGINALLY I'D BOUGHT THE BED for another girlfriend, the one before C. She'd insisted I get a king-size, one with enough space to guarantee a good night's sleep, one where she could lay on her back, her arms crossed over her chest in a death pose, insurance against my slow creeping during the night to slide my hand under her pillow, happy to feel the weight of her head through down and feather. I slept on the right side (as I do now with C.), the side nearest the bathroom, my path a sliver of wood floor and wall, the same tightrope walk I still make now in the dark, the wall to steady me as I negotiate dog-in-dog-bed, bench, rug, dresser, and door. Most nights I arrive at the bathroom unscathed, but others produce bruised ankles, calves, and tails. The bed is too big for the room, no question; the bed has been too big for every room it's ever been squeezed into.

In part, I am to blame. I chose an Eastern king, a choice only Californians must make when sizing up from a queen, the California king a longer (plus 4 inches) and narrower (minus 4 inches) bed than its Eastern counterpart, an implication we're taller and skinnier here in the Golden State, but more likely a product of our constant need to be original. I explained the difference to my girlfriend, the one before C., rattling the tape measure across the room so she could appreciate the extra width I was willing to sacrifice. She waved me off—unlike C., numbers were never her strong suit—and told me it was my bedroom, my house, so I should be the one to decide.

But the bed's size wasn't my girlfriend's only complaint. Noises, even small ones, would wake her. She would sit up, put in her earplugs, and announce she was signing off for the night. I waited until then to tell her things I was too scared to say when she could hear me. Once, just as she was falling asleep, I whispered, *I've been praying that you'll stay.* Her eyelids flickered, and for a moment I thought she'd heard me.

I picked out a new bed frame for the Eastern king, a simple platform style (no box spring, no footboard) made of solid American cherry in the Shaker tradition, all wood joinery, modest, utilitarian. Maybe this was the problem, rather than the size: such a plain bed was puritanical to the point of prudish. There were other choices, other woods, even upholstery, sleek European designs with matching nightstands that would have suited the small space. I had such a bed once, a wedding gift from my parents, the one I held onto after the divorce, a queen-size covered in black leather, with upholstered backrests that could be moved, slid in anywhere along the bed frame: at the head, as one would expect, for reading or watching TV; at the foot or sides when a hip needed support, or a thigh, or a pair of knees, clipped over the padded edge; and at those times when an angle needed opening or closing, raising or lowering, or whatever the case may be. This was the bed my girlfriend before C. found too confining, the bed I'd replaced with the Eastern king, and with its departure went the escapades and the experiments, the excitement of my prime.

Reason tells me lesbian bed death has nothing to do with the bed, but then again, we refer to our sexual history as whom we've *slept with* or (though somewhat dated) whom we've *bedded*, slang far tamer than the current *hit* or *tapped*, verbs that suggest an aggressive, adventurous spirit the bedroom cannot contain, terrain I'd explored (and hit and tapped) many times in my twenties, thirties, and even forties: the living room rug and the kitchen counter; the shower and the pool; the front and back seat; the park and the beach. Then the time comes when we want only a bed, a soft, ample plane to roam, foregoing the hard edges and sticky surfaces and itchy detritus of more exotic locations.

A few months ago, I went mattress shopping with my parents. We rode the escalator upstairs to Macy's home department and took turns stretching out on acres of pillow-tops. They refused my suggestion to move up to a king, worried they'd lose each other in so much space. For sixty-four years they have slept in the same queen bed, with its carved, velvet-paneled headboard and matching nightstands. If I spend the night at my parents' house, I tiptoe downstairs the next morning, gently knock on their door, and wait for my father's mumbling, the okay sign for me to poke my head in and find them on my mother's side, huddled in a heart, my father's arm draped over her shoulder.
A salesman finally approached us, our guide through the varieties of quilted damask, some filled with silk on one side, wool on the other—two sides for two seasons, spring and fall—and others with memory foam, a heat sensitive material that molds to the body, originally developed by NASA for its astronauts, the salesman emphasized, a detail meant to conjure a sense of floating, weightless, in the dark.

We spent our first night together, C. and I, in the living room, in front of a fire, on a sofa as deep as a twin bed (perhaps that's the answer). On our sides we just fit, face-to-face or nestled like spoons. And yet, I fell asleep on top of C., she my dense, muscled mattress, a living, breathing cushion for my long, bony frame, my head resting in the small triangle between her neck and shoulder, her arms around me, to save me from slipping to the floor. Just as I drifted off, I heard her whisper, *I hope this lasts.* Later, when I asked her what she meant, she denied saying anything.

Within a few months, the Eastern king became our bed. C. credits it for the best rest she's ever had. The mattress's latex core cradles our bodies, reducing pressure points, extinguishing friction and unnecessary heat buildup, the essentials to a healthy sex life quickly smothered by material too resilient, too accommodating. C. sleeps on her back and rarely moves; I roll side-to-side, plumping my three pillows to fill in the empty spaces, though there was a time when I, too, slept like the dead.

Latex also provides motion isolation by preventing the movement of one person from traveling across the mattress, potentially waking the other. The goal of motion isolation is to create harmony in the bedroom, similar to the contentment expressed by the couples featured in those late-night TV commercials for remote-controlled beds, with variable sleep numbers and articulated positions that cater to the individual's needs and desires. Motion isolation could explain why, when I reach for C. during the night, she rolls away onto her side, or when I lean over to kiss her while she's sleeping, she turns her head, almost involuntarily, with no trace of disturbance but for her softer snores. She never feels me get up during the night when I can't sleep, when I try to get to the bathroom unscathed, but if I wander across the mattress's vast, empty center to press against her warmth, her grumbles about my trespassing push me back to my side of the bed.

In the morning, C. asks me if I slept well. All else is forgotten. Perhaps if I had paid closer attention to the mattress's promise of isolation, I might not be where I am now.

Fortunately, the latex mattress has one considerable drawback: the impressions left by our motionless bodies, dips and depressions that can limit our natural movement, trapping us in the holes we dig while we sleep. To avoid this, C. and I keep to a quarterly schedule; it takes both of us to turn and flip the mattress in our earnest attempt to forestall the ruts we make for ourselves.

It's getting cold now, as cold as it gets in Southern California. I pull out the Dick and Jane flannel sheets my sister bought online for my birthday a few years ago—thick, white cotton printed with scenes from the storybooks of our childhood. The corners of the pillowcases are dog-chewed and frayed. I shake out the fitted sheet and turn it so Dick and Jane are right side up—playing hopscotch, eating ice cream, pulling a red wagon of puppies. Happy to be together. The pattern irritates me (as do the other sheets stacked in the linen cabinet—the sock monkeys and the cowboys and the three sets of polka dots), makes me wonder whether my tendency toward kitschy playfulness has gone too far, has ventured into territory best reserved for adulthood. A few years ago, when I suggested we buy more grown-up linens—organic cotton in colors like sea salt or pebble or rosewater—C. shook her head. I pressed her to explain, but she couldn't find words for her objection. I understood this reluctance, both hers and mine, as though the presence of such serious bedding might finally demand our serious attention.

Once I get the Dick and Jane top sheet even, I fold haphazard hospital corners and leave the rest untucked. I check a corner of the bed on C.'s side that has pulled apart, post from rail, a gaping half-inch exposing raw wood and double dowel joinery. The right thing to do would be to disassemble the whole lot: headboard, rails, and slats. It would take both of us to carry the Eastern king out, to navigate the tight corners down the hallway, through the living room, and out to the garage where C. has a work bench, fitted with a vise and a pegboard of tools. Normally, I can rely on C. to do the right thing. She knows how to fix things, how to follow directions. Anytime she catches me cheating, trying to cut corners in my chores around the house, she takes over and does the job herself—e.g., I am no longer allowed to do her laundry. So when I told C. about the bed, she promised she'd take a look at it. But that was months (maybe years) ago.

If we wait any longer, collapse will be inevitable. No bed can stand on three feet. I dig into my closet. Way in the back is an old wooden clog—perfect for a hammer. I start banging on the post to close the gap. Just as I get one dowel in, the other pops out. I chase the fracture back and forth, beating at it whack-a-mole style, leaving

94

crescent-shaped dents in the golden cherry. Finally, I throw down the clog. I lie down on C.'s spot on our clean Dick and Jane sheets. I give up. I'm done hammering.

CARINE TOPAL

BATHING IN THE HOT SPRINGS, ESALEN, 2008

I was naked from the start showering among strangers against a backdrop of ocean and sky, strangers who held nothing back when dropping their towels to step foot into the baths. Though my muscles relaxed and my blood vessels widened, I smelled like a cocktail of rheumatic healing, a pale mammal going white in sulfur and brine. One blond Adonis stood at the neck of the pool legs crossed penis dangling like a folded lily. I could not help but turn to look at it. When I'd had enough of him I turned again to look at the sea pressured on three sides by the bluffs of Big Sur. I promised I'd write about this: the sharp palisades edged into the Pacific, the moon hanging low in the night. And when I turned away from the moon I'd come to tell about, he was gone, and only his wet footprint remained, proof that such beauty existed.

JENNIFER LAGIER

AARP BOOTY CALL

Camille meets Roy at Applebee's
for an Early Bird Dinner.
They connected online at SeniorPeople.com,
found each other's profile intriguing.
Enjoyed "before" and "after" photos,
battle wounds of aging.

Both still have their own teeth,
a sense of humor,
raging libidos.
Qualify for AARP discounts
at restaurants, motels.
Love to eat, drink and travel.

After more dates,
they share a bed, discover
they can laugh at arthritic hips,
stretch marks, sagging boobs,
Cialis and wrinkles.

All that's missing
is flexibility, stamina,
nothing yoga can't cure.

BREAD

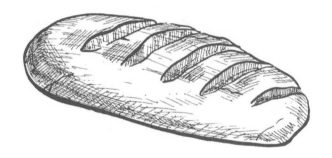

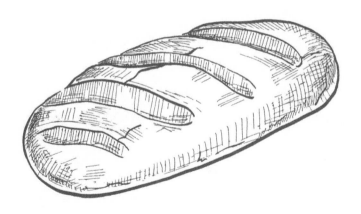

(sustenance)

ALEXIS RHONE FANCHER

VENUS IN SCORPIO

WHEN I WAS ALMOST FIFTY, single, and hornier than I'd ever been, a friend suggested I join match.com. It was time to find that illusive "Mr. Right," instead of settling for "Mr. Right Now."

I'd always had great sex. According to my astrologer, it was right there, in my chart. Multiple planets in Scorpio, he told me, including the sex planet, Venus. I'd survived two brief marriages in my twenties, both predicated on great sexual chemistry rather than real-life compatibility. I'd romped my way through my thirties and forties. Sexual pleasure, with both men and women, was a series of semi-serious, serially monogamous relationships that invariably fizzled out. This time, I was determined to find my *beshert* (destined one), a man of substance *and* sexual prowess.

I polished my match.com profile, and took the plunge: "Romantic Novelist Seeks True Life Hero," I wrote. "My cool exterior hides a passionate heart. Only the extraordinary need apply. He will not be disappointed."

Two weeks later, I met a guy. Tall, with fantastic blue eyes, Jim's audacious response to my profile had intrigued me: "I don't

101

think you look cool," he'd written. "I think you look hot. I *am* the extraordinary man you seek."

Our first date, lunch at the Sagebrush Cantina, segued into dinner that night. We couldn't get enough of each other. We had much in common, a love of theater and film, a lust for travel —a penchant for Beethoven's 9th Symphony. Even more important, we had similar values when it came to money, politics, sex and religion. Still, I was cautious, and dated a host of others who followed up on my profile; a Hollywood producer, a doctor from Bel Air, a litigation lawyer, a personal trainer, a retired coroner, a pilot, and the CEO of a Fortune 500 company.

But I was stuck from the first on Jim, that sweet, easy-going, "extraordinary" guy with an Ivy League education, the sonorous voice of a radio announcer, and a great sense of humor. He had an easy sexuality about him that I liked. Still, we took our time getting to know each other. We didn't jump into a sexual relationship. Rather, we let a friendship evolve first. Three months into dating, he blindfolded me on my birthday and drove us up the coast to a house on the beach, filled with all my favorite things; yellow roses, champagne, lobster. Everywhere there were silver balloons that said "I Love You" in big red letters. When we fell into bed with each other, we *made love*. And it was magical.

With two, high-powered careers, we had to *make time for sex*. Jim drove from his house to mine each morning at 5 a.m. We made love until 6:30, when he returned to his day, and I to mine. We saw each other whenever possible. We were married two years later.

We still make love every day. We purposely schedule it into our daily activities. We are flirtatious and often mistaken for newlyweds, even after fourteen years of marriage. It is about commitment and intent. My husband made it clear from the beginning that he is a man with a healthy sexual appetite. He told me that on his match. com profile he had found a way to "filter out" the 92 percent of women who didn't enjoy sex, who either "pretended to like it, or avoided sex altogether." I thank my lucky stars that I'm part of the remaining 8 percent. I wouldn't have it any other way.

A few months back, my husband and I hit a small rough patch. He felt neglected. I was finishing a poetry manuscript. It consumed me. My husband felt that making love with him had become an afterthought, and decided to withhold sex until he believed I had my priorities straight. It didn't take long. Day 1, I sailed through my day alone, making extraordinary progress on my manuscript. Day 2, when I reached for Jim, he hugged me, then turned away. Day 3, I no longer felt beautiful, desirable. I longed for his touch. I quickly realized what a huge place his affection had in my life, how I had taken daily sex, and the flirting and cuddling that came before and after, that filled my day with pleasure, for granted. I missed him and *it*, desperately. We had a heart-to-heart. No, my husband assured me, he wasn't angry. Withholding his physical affection for the better part of a week was just his way of showing me the error of my ways. That afternoon, when I jumped his bones, it was in lusty appreciation.

If we're fortunate, we get what we want in life, what we value. Our physical intimacy fuels our marriage. My man's touch thrills me, even after all these years. Still, he swears he married me for my mind. Go figure....

LESLIE ANNE MCILROY

FRENCH KISSING AT FIFTY

I didn't think I'd get old.
So imagine me startled
when I am not famous
and have not had sex
in a year, my fiftieth
birthday, another day,
shoulder frozen so I
can't reach anymore,
or swing or hit.

It happens, the doctor says,
to people your age. Therapy/
heat/ice/tramadol. I flap
my arms like a cartoon bird
practicing for takeoff three
times a day, hoping for give.

I know it is crazy to kiss
post-fifty, and the young
men with their hair are just
dreams, but if I could move
my arm, maybe I could wave
that boy down, motion something
come hither, like the backing-up
of a truck, gesture wide enough
to let him in, maybe

I could use my tongue.

Liz Rose Dolan

Still

I like to watch
him turning his head
as wisps of hair lick his thick neck.

I like to watch him pull off his specs
when he really needs to see
and toss them into the back seat
before he rubs his scruffy beard
against my cheek.
Just rough enough
so I can still feel it chafing
before I sleep. Still I like to watch

as he laces his boots
that flaunt his sturdy legs
watch his hips sway
as he pumps iron
to U2's *With or Without You.*

When he speaks I don't
hear a word
so entranced am I by
the up and down motion
of his square jaw
the lilt of his full lips.

Standing behind him I run my fingers
from his bronzed shoulders to his ticklish waist
press the curve of my lap against his ass.

He's my aeolian harp, my tin whistle, my bodran.
Without him I'd be a cold, silvery night
full of shivers and empty promise.

Lisa Rizzo

The Single Woman: The Other Side

HERE IS THE THING: I'm tired of explaining why I'm single and doing nothing to change my state. Except for a brief two-year marriage, I've been single since I was thirty. Thirty years of no serious relationships, just a few dates and flirtations, one disastrous personal ad experience (back in the old days before online dating when you found those ads in the back of newspapers among ones for hot, nude girls). But other than those, no romantic relationships at all.

For years I wondered what was wrong with me: too much feminism, not enough fatherly love, laziness, fear? When asked, I made the excuse that my marriage had burned away all interest in love. And in some way that is true. After a five-year depression from a divorce made worse by continuing to be involved with my ex-husband (stupidly, I admit), I just didn't want a relationship anymore. The last straw was a messy night with the Ex on my thirtieth birthday. I said enough is enough.

At first it wasn't simple to renounce romantic involvement. Everyone wanted to know how I felt about it. My friends and family were concerned about me. My father said it must be that I hate men.

A co-worker, a lesbian, asked, "Why don't you try women?" My "I did," shut her up.

Another colleague told me about successfully meeting her husband while hanging out at the bar of the yacht club. "You have to play the game," she said. I replied, "I play my own game." And that is exactly what I wanted.

Dinner parties often included some form of the Let's Quiz Lisa game from well-meaning friends and curious acquaintances. *Why aren't you married? Why aren't you trying to find someone? How do you feel about this? Are you happy?* I cheerfully answered all the questions, putting on a brave face. But underneath it all, I knew what they were really asking: What's *wrong* with you?

Don't get me wrong. I'm not opposed to marriage. I have lots of married friends. All my siblings are married. My parents have been married for more than sixty years. I cry at wedding ceremonies. I think it's wonderful for those people. Just not for me.

The plain fact of the matter is that I just don't care enough about having a man to try to get one. I am happy being single. I am not just resigned or adjusted to it. I haven't had to come to terms with my singlehood as a strange path my life took. At sixty, I can finally embrace the realization that I actually chose to remain single. Perhaps at first it was unconscious, but I have come to accept that I made this choice. There, I've come out.

I'm not alone in this. The word has gotten out. According to the U.S. Census, for the first time ever, single adult women outnumber married adult women in the United States. We're becoming famous. Rebecca Traister has even written a book about us: *All the Single Ladies*.

Even so, Traister couldn't quite keep from making excuses for us. In an interview with NPR's *Fresh Air* host, Terry Gross, she said, "The choice not to marry isn't necessarily a conscious rejection of marriage. It is [about] the ability to live singly if an appealing marriage option doesn't come along." This sounds like the explanations I once gave to people.

As a single woman, I need to stand up for myself. There are good reasons to stay single. Unlike women with partners, I don't have to negotiate with someone about where to go for vacation, what shows to watch or going to see in-laws. Quite frankly, the best thing about being single is not having in-laws. My time is all mine to figure out how to spend it. I travel where I want to go and do not need to fight for alone time.

Still, how does a woman in her sixties survive in a world where she is constantly bombarded by images of young women in sexy clothes (or not) on magazine covers? In a world where even Susan Sarandon claims that the way she stays young looking is by having sex? I'm not a prude or shriveled up. I think sex is great. But is constant availability absolutely necessary for my happiness and wellbeing? Many people in our society think so, but I don't believe it.

In the last half of my life, I've decided to focus on complete sensuality rather than only sexuality. We equate physicality with sex and so we ignore or downplay all the other wonderful physical pleasures the world has to offer us. I refuse to do that. I value hugs from friends or kisses from nieces and nephews, even friends' dogs. I revel in the pleasure of a hot tub or the cold salt water from ocean waves. All offering sensual satisfaction.

But what about love, you might ask? There too I have an abundance: wonderfully loving relationships with siblings and parents, sisters and brother-in-laws, my niece who is the love of my life. And deep, satisfying relationships with friends. Enough love to keep me warm for the rest of my life.

One of the good things about getting older has been the dwindling away of those questions. After I turned fifty, people spent less time trying to figure me out. By fifty-five, I was just seen as a confirmed old maid, a spinster, the maiden aunt. I became invisible, no longer seen as sexually viable. Other women might mourn this indication of society's prejudice against older women, but for me it was a relief. I could stop explaining myself and get on with my own happy life.

I'm fortunate to have met many older single women who are my mentors and role models. One of those friends told me: "At first I was lonely. Then the loneliness turned into a beautiful solitude." Those are words I live by.

DIANA RAAB

TWO WORLDS

Let's live in two worlds
the way lovers do
the way we should
the one we face every day,
littered with family goings on
and work affairs and then
let me gently meander over to your world
the world of great imaginations,
travels to untouched venues
sleeping in beds never opened
holding hands in foreign streets
walking new mountains
tasting sweet foreign foods
all while gazing into those
deep brown bedroom tunnels
which always tell me they want me,
sometimes slits, sometimes
wide open in amazement
at the pleasures
my lips bring to yours.

Where did you come from
and please don't tell me
that you will ever go.

Promise?

BECKY DENNISON SAKELLARIOU

UNREPENTANT BODY

I walk days without another's touch, keeping
desire braided tight. My skin moults,
liquid seeping to the raw surface.

I could loose it all upon
this raging world, race through the market,
run my palms down the naked chest of the fish monger

as I turn from the gray marble slab and pay.
What is a body for? ready, wanting another body
to lie across, to fold into, to do what humans long to do.

A woman like me is invisible, if she is not,
she should be, an anathema, a sin.
My grandmother kept her whole body

covered, no *want* in her vocabulary,
my mother didn't know how
to want, my sister wanted, telling no one.

A bathtub, clean hands, wet fingers
run down the arm, touch the neck,
pause at the damp skin under the breast.

The women in the Turkish *hammam*
appalled at my pubic hair, mimic shaving,
shake their heads disapprovingly, *tsou tsou.* Dirty hair.

I can see that they too yearn,
their thin singlets wet against their skin,

breasts and thighs soaked in suds,
Eve, her sisters, her mother, loving,

longing, washing each other, washing
the dead, in this, their precious House

before God came and decided otherwise.

Carolyn Butcher

Touch Me

What makes the engine go?
Desire, desire, desire.
The longing for the dance
stirs in the buried life.
One season only,
  and it's done.
So let the battered old willow
thrash against the windowpanes
and the house timbers creak.
Darling, do you remember
the man you married? Touch me,
remind me who I am.

—Stanley Kunitz, 1905-2006

Around the time of my fiftieth birthday, I had my birth chart analyzed by an experienced astrological consultant who knew nothing about me. I was untroubled in my life, but curious at how and where I stood at my half-century. In excellent health but with a family history of death before age seventy-five, I was beginning to ask myself how I would like to spend the remaining years of my life. I remember being deliberately, and uncharacteristically, quiet as I sat down in the astrologer's office. She had laid my chart out on a coffee table beside a cassette recorder. I was determined not to say or do anything that would give away any information about myself. After telling me that my sun sign, Virgo, is ruled by Mercury, and explaining the intellectual influence of that planet, the astrologer said I had "a chart par excellence of a writer and actually what would be your best use of it, if you chose, would be literary criticism—and I do not know what you do."

At the time I was writing my Ph.D. dissertation on James Joyce's *Finnegans Wake*.

She had me, in less than five minutes.

The astrologer was particularly interested in the overwhelming dominance of Mars, whose strong sexual energy was not connected with the rest of my chart and could therefore "lead you in the wrong place sometimes." When I assured her I had been faithful to the same man for twenty-nine years, her surprised response asked, "Well, I wonder how you managed that?" I told her my husband was comfortable with my having male friends with whom I interacted within very clear boundaries. It was an honest attempt to make sense of my life and she commended me on an amazing accomplishment, "given your chart." Now I look at what I thought was a completely plausible answer with tenderness and compassion toward the woman I am no longer. Later, after my astrologer became my psychotherapist, we began the long journey to an understanding that my explanation on that afternoon was the first evidence of a protective mask that concealed my unmet, even unacknowledged, emotional desires and needs.

My physical needs were well covered. While I was nearly always the instigator, my husband was a willing sexual playmate. Lock the automatic gates so we could make love mid-afternoon on a blanket on the lawn? Oh the joys of the kids being away at college. A hotel room in a former palace with the windows open to the Grand Canal in Venice? This is what we have money for. Is the Jacuzzi tub in our new bathroom big enough for two? You betcha. Another woman might have left the astrological reading that afternoon with a license to fool around, feeling that the sexual cards she had been dealt at the moment of her birth made fighting adultery impossible. I left on a smug cloud, congratulating myself not only on the strength of my ethical and moral standards as a loyal wife, but also on how clever, creative and honorable I was in my relationships with men.

I tapped my husband for sex as soon as I returned home that afternoon. But five years later I was divorced and married to one of those male friends with whom the boundaries had fallen away.

Fifteen years have passed since that meeting with the astrologer, and as I look back it would be tempting to credit (or blame) the reading of my birth chart for the changes in my life. But, I do not think I was the only woman at mid-life at the turn of the millennium who was taking a peek at the world beyond my protective mask and asking, *Is this all there is?* Those of us who were born in the early 1950s are too young to have been at the vanguard of the sexual revolution and yet we are old enough to have grown up with the traditional expectation that our personal and financial security could only be secured through marriage. Almost all the women I know who are my age were married before they were twenty-four; some of them in high-waisted wedding dresses concealing their three- or four-month baby bumps.

Having grown up as a child in post-war England, I felt the communal angst of insecure survival. Picnics at the beach always began with a reminder to us children (as we clutched our buckets and spades) never to touch anything metal in the sand because it could be an un-exploded bomb. Our parents, in their turn, had been born within a decade of the end of the First World War. An entire generation of potential husbands had been wiped out, leaving the social, financial and political problem of two million "Surplus Women" in Britain.

These were the older nuns teaching us in the convent schools and the maiden aunts of our mothers and fathers. The word "spinster" was still on government forms as a choice to explain a woman's marital status; an ugly word with terrifying implications of either poverty or lifetime dependency on male family members. As a result, there remained an anxiety within British society regarding unsupported women, and so our parents congratulated their friends (who breathed a sigh of relief) when their daughters became engaged.

However, we were living lives beneath the parental radar. While nice girls did not discuss sex even among themselves, the availability of the birth control pill from family planning clinics or from GPs (in order to treat "menstrual problems") meant there was no longer a fear of pregnancy. We understood that losing our virginity was a performance of some sort of freedom. But freedom from what? Freedom to do what? Cool girls walked around with a copy of Sylvia Plath's *The Bell Jar* under their arms because its possession symbolized a self-awareness of disorientation with society's expectations of what they were supposed to do with their lives. But in the end, after a few years of work or university, and maybe one or two sexual partners, young women happily became wives and mothers.

My birth chart suggests that in my growing-up years my emotional needs were invisible, with no veracity of their own, but I suspect this would be mirrored by most girls of my era. We were taught from an early age to mask our needs and therefore our desires, and any unmasking took a great deal of work. For most of us that did not happen until our Chiron return at the age of fifty, when the stars were aligned once again as they were at the moment of our birth, and we were dealt the opportunity for a mulligan, a do-over. Some women could not take advantage of that opportunity for financial reasons or because of familial duties or societal pressures. Some were too fearful. But I could and I did.

At the age of twenty-two I had made a good marriage, married the right man, become a good wife, who in return was well provided for. But at fifty-two I was no longer that woman and I was acutely aware of a sensual gulf that I could not bridge and in which I did not want to spend the remaining years of my life. After the decision to end our thirty-year marriage was final, my husband and I moved into a surreal relationship. There was a raw-to-the-bone tenderness in our interactions and a desperately affectionate calm about the house where we both still lived. I don't remember such nitty gritty details as whether I cooked meals for two, but I do know that we still slept in the same bed and even continued to have sex—although that had morphed into a desperately sad coupling of confirmation that the "there" really wasn't there any more. I was overwhelmed with a yearning that became clear in an extraordinary dream I recorded in my journal:

It is the day of a trial and I am extraordinarily happy—elated even. The building where the trial is taking place is like a theatre. Big, heavy, wooden double doors open to a street that is unfamiliar to me. I can see through to the outside and it is bright and sunny. A happy busy town.

Inside the building there is a carnival atmosphere, like Mardi Gras. I am having a great time. My husband isn't there; I am expecting him and can't wait to share this with him because it is so bizarre. The judge is a voluptuous woman wearing a costume with a headdress and mask, which she removes frequently—in other words, she is not hiding behind it. The crowd is there to see her. She is spectacularly funny, very entertaining, and yet she commands the respect of everyone. She is considered highly intelligent, fair, sees through bullshit, intuitive, totally connected.

At one point, the judge's pet goose wanders through a crowd with her goslings surrounding her. The ground is dirt, and she does not seem out of place. The goose is supposed to be there; in fact her entrance was expected by the crowd. I am so happy, completely caught up in what is going on around me; trying hard not to miss anything. In the back of my mind I am thinking: Where is my husband? He is missing this and it is so much fun.

My husband arrives in a dark suit, although when I see him from the rear he is wearing his tan waterproof jacket. He can't find me and I can't get to him because of the enormous number of people. But he seems unaware of what is going on around him and I realize with disappointment that he is not going to have the same reaction as me. He doesn't "get" it.

I go outside for a break—my senses are overly stimulated.

I find a quiet corner in the sunny garden under a small tree. Suddenly I hear a bird, and its song sounds as if it is saying, "I am starving." I search and find a large, gray bird. It is fluttering around, desperate and crying, "I am starving." I see that its beak has been sawn off. It tries to peck at me, but it can't hurt because of its damaged beak. I give it some cold slices of beef. It is still desperate and saying, "I am starving," and I feed it everything I can find: bugs, garbage, anything. It is so hungry and I can't bear to hear it saying, "I am starving."

After a while, the bird settles down and we begin to talk (yes… the bird and I). Now the bird's beak looks different. Although too short, it has been sanded and shaped into something approximating a beak. I ponder what to do with it, because I don't want a pet bird. I say I will look after it until I can get it to a bird rescue place where they will find a good home for him (yes, the bird is male). He says he is owned by a guy named Bob. I ask how the bird sleeps at night. What will he need? He tells me he needs a medium-thin dowel on which to perch for sleeping just large enough for its claws to hang on to. For the daytime, he will need a larger dowel on which to sit.

I wrote in the journal that I thought I was probably both the judge and the bird.

Meanwhile, my needs had been recognized. My friend and I were sitting in my car listening to a baseball game, having arrived too early for a showing of a documentary about Jacques Derrida. I felt an electrical charge in the air and I leaned over to kiss him because I wanted to know what it would feel like. He was one of my best friends in graduate school and, although he had not been in my thoughts romantically, apparently the same was not true for him. After the kiss, he said: "I love you, and I've loved you for four years. I've been watching you and I know how sad you have been. You need someone to love you and take care of you and to make love to you—and I'm the one."

I said, "Not here, not now..." and he smiled and said, "No, of course not. You just tell me when you are ready and I will make it special."

Then we went into the movie and as soon as the lights went down he picked up my hand and stroked the inside of my forearm lightly as a feather for the next ninety minutes. The following day, I telephoned him and told him I was ready. In his bed a few days later, my tears once more flowed uncontrollably at the moment of orgasm but, unlike the last few years with my husband, this time it was because the voids in my heart and my soul had been filled. And this man noticed and held me and stroked my hair until the tears stopped. Then he got out of bed and came back a few minutes later with a mug of tea and oatmeal cookies he had baked that morning.

Twelve years later we are married and he still brings me tea in bed.

Sometimes he doesn't bother to get dressed first.

At sixty-five, I have no greater joy than being brought a mug of tea by a naked man who touches me and reminds me who I am.

Eileen Malone

Jacaranda

Overturn your wheelbarrow
full of pale-purpled damp jacaranda leaves
lie down with me, naked, here in the garden's
morning of raspberry drizzle

between fresh worms rooting in yeasting earth
among the rosy fragrance of fallen apples
broken to reveal their cores, their stars of seeds
flood me, bury me in strawberry and lake water

give me your lips, kiss me in amaranth, jasmine
open your mouth with its small startle of dark spikes
like shark teeth straining, let me swim to you
surrender to the current

let us peel away this false dawn from dappled things
bejangled roots, ferny, riffled leaflight, as I embrace
your naked waist on a bed of purple leaves up from
this lush pile of the jacarandas' lavender snow
a crush, a compost mulch of now, of all that is left
of what once was early.

HAIDEN FAIRLY

SEX IN CAPTIVITY

When my husband wants me,
he gets quiet and alert.
His senses all fine-tuned, ears pricked for exquisite listening.
He watches me from across the room,
I know the look, attentive to my every move.
I am caught in his visual snare;
he a predator watching his prey.
But he is a domesticated animal, and will do my bidding.
The toilet needs cleaning?
He trots off with a wire brush to do the deed,
his cock leading the way,
penis overriding normal brain functions.
When the toilet's clean, I want to talk.
I demand his undivided attention, and remarkably,
he listens. Words hang between us.
A delicate curtain laced with expectation.
Soon he pushes aside the fabric of conversation.
Presses onto me, inside of me.
An urgent desire takes hold.
I arch like a stroked cat.
Sensations ripple across my back.
He massages me, kisses me, licks me,
nibbles me. Strokes my hair.
I give myself to him,
as I always do.
The hunt is over, the dance begins.

Tania Pryputniewicz

Sex, Hammers, and Self-care in a House with Three Children

FROM WHERE I'M LODGED under my husband, sunlight streaming across our torsos, I can hear the kids in the yard with hammers. Though we've given them goggles to wear for this latest rock-crushing obsession, I thought we'd said to them: *Parents Present or No Go*. On a "honey-I'm-home-from-work-early" high, my husband is voting for tuning their voices out, which I'm convinced he must have a special gene for, while I, at the opposite end of the spectrum, suffer from full libido lockdown. How romantic, I think, were I a husband to such a woman, whose post-coital refrain might as well be, "Can I get up now?"

I'm thinking of the Sigourney Weaver article in a More magazine I read earlier at the dentist's office. Weaver describes her screen test for "Alien," which included "a scene that's not in the movie where the Captain and Ripley have sex. I said to Ridley [director Scott], 'That is so ridiculous...'"—and here I got called by the dentist, but to paraphrase and finish her sentence, *Who could possibly think about*

123

sex with that monster on the loose? Like I said, for me, it's not so much a god-forsaken-motorboat-headed-monster oozing oil from his row of metal remote-control teeth that is the libido killer, but the kids... the sound of their voices, second only to the sound of my mother-in-law's voice or the voices of other people's children on sleepovers.

We persevere, until I can no longer deny that I'm burning internally. Which at first seemed like not a bad thing...but I mean, *burning.* "Something's wrong," I say to my husband, to which he cocks his head to the window for a moment, and replies, "No one is crying, they're fine." "No," I say, "I mean, with me." Then I remember yesterday at the health club, finally getting to an hour of "self-care," I'd sunk down into the swirling hot tub, the air above the water a cross between halitosis and dirty socks.

I said to the woman across from me, "Do you smell that?" To which she replied, "Yeah, but it's better than the slime that was in the corner of the tub yesterday." I got out immediately, made a note to tell the staff, showered, and forgot all about it.

Clearly the source of the burning. Given the seven-day regime of sticky Monostat snow, I've switched allegiances to the steam room. Where the sound of the steam filling the room and the way it narrows my vision makes me wonder if I've prematurely added the pressure of "relaxing and getting in shape" to my list of things to do on the way to putting myself together in order to—now that two out of three kids are launched—*Getting a Real Job* instead of *Just Taking Care of the Kids.*

At the dinner table that night, my husband and I notice a green/blue egg on our middle son's forehead. He and his sister drop their eyes when we ask about it, further confirming our suspicions that a cover-up is under way as they silently eat all the carrots on their plates. "He...uh...did it to himself," says my daughter. "Yeah," says my son, "by accident. It doesn't hurt, I swear, Mom." The littlest will spill the beans the next day, you can count on him to crack: he was swinging the hammer and didn't see his brother's head (doing little to convince me that sex while the kids are awake is ever a decent plan, as I've said oh-so-many times).

My husband waves such evidence aside with his carpe-diem approach to life, and takes more delight in their collusion: "Aw honey, look, they're ganging up on us. Isn't that cute?" I gather up the hammers and tuck them as far away as possible in the garage. Back upstairs, I leave a voicemail for the maintenance guy at the club, stumbling over the phrase, "gynecological problem," and forgetting to leave my name. I hesitate, consider calling back, then stop. *Why,* I convince myself, *would he need to call me back anyway...for proof?*

CATHIE SANDSTROM

LOVE AT THIS AGE

Breast to breast, we are two
mature nations discovering
a common frontier one person wide.

That first morning, light over the transom
lit and back-lit the white hair on your chest.
How you lay on your back, eyes closed in

intimate communion. So much falls away—
lifting to the surface, your sacred beauty.
In this room shot through with vectors

of light, our mirrored ghosts reflected
in a glassed frame, insubstantial,
unhurried. A new kind of acceptance.

In the restaurant as you walk away,
the hem of your jacket, hiked slightly
over forward-rolled shoulders,

unnoticeable from the front. We are still
vulnerable. After the marriages, the conflicts
and uncertainties, the years of waiting,

still   vulnerable.

Diane Kimball

The Bed, the Carpet, and the Jeep

I

NARROW AND MUSTY with age, the stairwell wound up four floors to the *atelier*, to our Paris magic. The tiny room under the eaves. The view over the city. The bed, scrumptious. At least it probably was. Yikes! I can't remember if the sheets were white and the pillows down. You see, that was twenty years ago; I struggle to recoup the intensity from that time. I was divorced and about to turn fifty. He was younger, a lover, a fellow musician who was married to someone else far away in America. I recognized in him a haven, a harbor of romance and risk.

Romance was defined in a glass of wine on a quiet street on the *Ile St. Louis*. In a dinner of *steak frites* served in a modest restaurant along the Seine. In a view of Notre Dame from the window of our room. He was the knight and I...well, I certainly was no maiden. And that's the better part. Older, you know how to give...to receive...to make *love*. Such is the, shall I call it *mythical?*, narrative that we girls-to-women read in Arthurian legends. Well, how could I not have fallen for the story? Actually, I fell *into* the story. Interpreting the *ideal* of courtly love into my own experience. I called him *Mon Lion*, my lion. I, his *Gazelle*.

We're here in Paris for a week. We make love in the evenings. The only danger I see is that I still have periods and he is potent. Careful and cautious about this, I use a spermicide and the requisite KY lubricant. Not narrow and musty with age yet! We are together, away from people, at least those we know. Away from work, from phones, from interruptions. It's the late 1990s and Paris is safe and secure. For us, for our moments together.

The knight and his lady, this friend and I, hiked up into the Eiffel Tower. Earning a glimpse of what became for me, at that moment in my life, the sublime.

> *and the sands in the glass*
> *stopped*
> *for a pure white moment*
> *while gravity sprinkled upward*
> —Mary Oliver

II

We meet during the final era of the personal ads. 2002. We're in Barnes and Noble, probably in the sale book section. Laughing. He has a French background and nose to match. I am teaching French in a neighborhood middle school. I am hoping for honesty. He tells me he's had kidney cancer. His world, his reality. I will choose to step into it. We're both fifty-seven.

He's jovial, joyous even, a spontaneous friend and soon, lover. He's a widower and a surgeon, a retired urologist. Kind of funny, I think. He knows women's…well, systems.

"I've heard about the older woman's *unopposed* testosterone," he remarks after our first lovemaking.

"And what do you think about that?" I feel unabashedly alive. "We could support those statistics…"

He laughs and I know he is happy. What neither of us knows, or cares about, is time. Time left. The death of life is hanging out like a sloth, never intruding, at least for months. We travel, explore, enliven each other's lives. We glimpse an eagle in Alaska's Prince William Sound, a moray eel in the waters of Bonnaire, a brilliant orange sky over Lake Michigan. Our lovemaking becomes urgent. He tells me he's never had oral sex. I delight him the first time, and the next, and the next. Is this a wave we're riding? We're out at sea, drifting. And willing. I name his expansive condo on a grassy hill *le chateau*. He is *Monsieur Boucheron*, from the brand of his favorite aftershave. We're packing ten years into an unknown number of months.

He greets me at the door in a beret and penciled-on French moustache. I expose a partial breast for him and he accepts. Soon he's exquisitely carving the grilled chicken with the skill and grace of his trade.

"So that's how you do it!" I suggest.

"No, we'll wait till later to find out," he whispers.

His "later" means the den. In front of the fireplace. On the carpet.

Well, I can't say that I'm all that comfortable. I like to roll over, be on my belly, and get aroused that way. The floor is hard and the carpet scratchy. Maybe he's had a good time. He certainly came easily. I'm working on it…

He guides me, supports my decision to retire, and loves me intensely. He, this man, a gift to me. Offering me the privilege to be at his side, in his bed, at his death. I begin to realize that he's done. He's invited the peripheral angels into his vision. And I can't do a damn thing about it.

"I've heard it's the first thing to go," he says.

We, unknowingly, have a week to go. Fuck. Why am I thinking we could have one last, lasting lovemaking? Then I let all that go.

Late August morning. Michigan humid heat, birds in gaudy dress. A tall bedroom window opened slightly to the dogwoods below. He is propped on pillows on the altar-white sheets of his bed. The bed where we've played as vibrant lovers.

Early afternoon. Clouds have dusted the sky with a soft billow of down. His breath rasps, pauses. Then begins again. I'm in front of him, watching his eyes.

"It's okay to let go. I love you very much." I kiss the whisper into his ear.

Late afternoon. The soft light rests only on him. His last breath, ending. I ease my hands, slowly, under his head and his legs. I feel a vibration, a quiet resonance of him. And of what I call Spirit. Slivers of dusk light have scattered over every atom in the bedroom. And yet, there is still room to breathe.

I am not expecting death. I am expecting to cross it, to spend it.
—Hélène Cixous

III

Last year I turned seventy. How can this be? I have tons of energy, ideas, and opinions. I have one less kidney. Not in the plan I had about my health. It had to be taken out to determine that, in a 3 percent probability, the tumor was benign. I have both breasts, still beautiful, actually larger due to what I call *wine-weight*. Less pubic hair, a regret! I'm Anglo-Canadian-American, fair-haired with a vibrant Celtic heritage. I know that's where the full pubic bush came from. And still filled with a *wanderlust* that has to be female, full-blooded DNA stuff. Menopause, now a long gone issue. Yikes! My oldest granddaughter is turning twenty-three. Gotta' live it now!

Wait! A thousand sunsets? Uncountable intimate moments? An eternity of this human intimacy…sex? Read the statistics: women and men who knew each other, earlier, once, long ago, reconnecting in older age. Spouses have died, divorced, are long gone. A *now* place to inhabit with wisdom and grace. Here I go again. He's this, my traveling buddy. He hides a paunch under Aloha shirts and a balding head under a baseball cap. A widower. I've known him since 1986. We taught kids together. We've been in those middle school trenches. We've got history. We feel comfortable with each other. We'll write our own adventures on the sands of Waikiki Beach, in a hot air balloon in Cappadocia, on a golf course (Ouch! senior stereotype) in Jasper.

And in Madrid. 2015. We discover the theater district on a late night, high July heat near the Plaza Major. We've had an afternoon romp through Madrid's archeological museum. Later, delicious tapas in a decidedly *locales* bar. Romance. Spanish style. *Muy rica!* We make love in our ultra-modern hotel room at 2 a.m. Okay, so in Spain he's *Bruno*. You can guess the connection to *un toreador.*

We begin to call these moments…*Seniors Gone Wild!* You see, it doesn't have to be Paris. Or Madrid. Sometimes you just want to have sex in your own back yard.

October requires a campfire when you live in Michigan. In the woods. We pull out the canvas chairs, pour a glass of wine, poke the fire. We talk about teachers today who get no respect, about us seniors who get no increase in Social Security, about humpback whales whose breeding grounds are threatened by warming oceans. The line between serious and comical blurs. Oh, yes! We've been around that proverbial block.

He disappears for a bit. I hear a car engine. He's backing the jeep up to the fire. Inside a sleeping bag, rolled out. I've never done this before. Let's do it! Wait! I have to run inside to get the older woman's life-saving (Calendula-Thuja) vag-gel. I bet he's taken his pill. Soon, I'm in the back, on my back, feet touching the top of the jeep. I'm laughing so hard; can he get inside me? He's there, I'm there, we're there, wherever there is. I'm seventy. He's seventy-three.

This time of year, the autumn, calls in the beginning of the end. At older age, the path, the places, unfold still. Unique and common. Unrepeatable, yet known. Intimacy, connection, and pure, lovely sex. From one eternity to another. Or rather, up one stairway...

One...has seen a thousand sunsets, each unique and unrepeatable...
—William Martin

IRENE FICK

SEX ON THE SAND

On the shallow slope of sixty, this slide
into old age, I wonder, in an idle way,
as we stroll along the water's edge,
what it would be like if we mustered up the grit
to have sex here on the sand, yes, sex
on the sand, before it's too late,

before we shrink, become another old pair,
two gray silhouettes curved over silver walkers
as we make careful passage down railed hallways
for the four o'clock serving where table talk starts,
stalls, then settles on portion sizes, ailing joints,
who will succumb to the cherry cheesecake?

Will we rue the day we turned down the chance to play
Burt and Deborah, find our own secret eternity
on the sands of the state park, where the waves pummel
the shoreline, where we would have unzipped, stripped,
sprawled on some illicit dune, flushed and breathless,
ignoring the sand needling our sweaty skin.

Well. This is how I imagine it. In truth,
sex on the sand is just a reckless notion, like sex
on the kitchen table, or sky-bound in the jet's lavatory,
or pinned to the walls of a high-rise elevator,
a titillating story to relish, shock old friends.

Now, on the shallow slope of sixty, our limbs
no longer stretch and straddle at will, prefer to lie
on a sleep-numbered mattress with clean cotton sheets.

For now, for us, the ceiling fan dispatches
a gentle breeze, the noise machine from K-Mart
whooshes ocean sounds, and the two of us sink,
as always, into a familiar pattern of flesh upon flesh,
a cushion for all that comes next.

FIGS

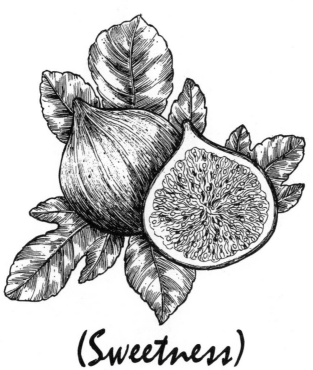

(Sweetness)

Eva Haller

Philemon and Baucis

Long, long ago on a high hill in Greece stood a beautiful linden tree, its branches intertwined with a mighty oak. The two trees were once Philemon and Baucis, two young lovers whose love was so strong, their life so gentle, that when it came time for their departure from this earth Zeus granted their wish, and turned them into these two magnificent trees.

My father often told me this story as I was falling asleep, and I remember how as a child I envisioned my parents' arms intertwined, walking down the Greek hill.

My father called my mother Baucis, and my mother, who was not a scholar of ancient legend, somewhat reluctantly and quietly called my father Philemon.

I lived my first eighteen years with this tender couple, learning acceptance, care and quiet sexuality. When my father became ill, my mother became a full-time nurse, and turned her love into devotion. They were a loyal couple.

So I learned about marriage from these intertwined trees, and it came into full use in my life's story.

I married an amazing man, larger than life, brilliant in every way. He loved me bigger than life, and he stretched me, giving me self-confidence, applauding my achievements, and giving me courage to be more than me.

And then he died.

Life was not much fun without him, and sex was not interesting with anyone else, though God knows I tried to hide my pain behind acting out sexually. Sex is no fun without joy. Sex is not a sport activity, nor is it a way to develop deep relationship. We humans need other forms of communication and understanding to accompany the act of love.

I remember bursting into tears when a kind man put his jacket on my shoulders at a dinner party one night. The awareness of each other's need is so important and meaningful.

Then, after a few years of frustrating widowhood I met a man who equally suffered the loss of the love of his life. We found joy in each other, because we had joy in our past partners.

Finding new love, and growing old together is simply wonderful. We are both eighty-seven years old, and enjoy love-making. Is it different than when we were younger? Oh, yes. There is gratitude, a huge portion of tenderness, a bit of fear, because what if we no longer have each other? Caressing an old body is softer, gravity has added its sculptural aspects, and the words accompanying sex are more about gratitude and appreciation.

It is so interesting to note that when one talks to young people about having a sex life, there often is embarrassment on their part. As if one should not or could not have sex after a certain age. There is no time limit for caring for each other. No physical reason to stop wanting one's mate.

Philemon and Baucis lived a very long time, they became stooped, wrinkled, forgetful, and each year they wanted more years to enjoy each other. The only request they had from Zeus was that they leave this earth together.

And so they did!

DAVI WALDERS

ANNIVERSARY

That you and I, I and you,
this twentyfifth year after
you stamped your foot, shattered
the glass, and friends, so many dead
or forgotten, applauded in a ballroom
long abandoned, twentyfive years
of Monday goodbyes, monthly wars
with stacks of bills, bags of garbage,
frozen gutters, nights filled
with pink medicines, fevered cheeks
on shoulders, the other hand reaching
for the pediatrician's call, termites
chewing, and hours waiting
for the door to open, holding
our own daughter's head vomiting
beer into our own leaking toilet,
that now, as mirrors mark the descent
of breasts, the tub catches silvered
hair and our eyes wear pouches
and hoods, as though expecting rain,
that you and I could smell the salt
of each other, coming together after
long absence, silent, still, staring up
at the darkening ceiling, naked in a house
with empty, orderly bedrooms, the last
of dead roses and discarded boyfriends
tossed out, your hand touching mine,
our breathing slowing,
the wonder of it all.

PAM DAVENPORT

THIS HASN'T HAPPENED YET AND NOW YOU'RE OLD BUT STILL

Your weathered skin,
your body bent
from years on horseback,
your thick hair
persisting across your head,
your crooked
overlapping teeth,
your sharp teeth in your
insatiable mouth,
I would like to offer
up my tender skin,
the inside of my upper arm,
my thigh my hip,
to your voracious teeth,
I want to let you tear at my flesh,
I want you to make me bleed.

Sally Franz

Tweaking Sex After Fifty

Sexually women got royally boinked when Hugh Hefner started boffing every bunny in his burrow. His message? Sex was okay with two consenting adults. The caveat? The woman had to have ginormous boobs, no brain, and be willing to expose herself for pay in a centerfold. The result was girls started dumbing down (even further) and anorexia and bulimia entered the medical dictionaries. But alas, it is impossible to compete with air brushing. Turns out being a "cherished/respected" plasticized Barbie doll means being objectified. If that makes women happy I don't think models would be pouting down the runway in-between bouts at the rehab center.

And a shout out to Disney. Someday the Prince will come, baby you, love you perfectly, pay for your every whim, and, of course, read your mind. You will fall into each other's arms and bluebirds will start chirping. Like the Little Mermaid, all it costs you is your authentic voice and soul.

Enter (so to speak) FREE LOVE and THE PILL. It meant screwing at will and never having to say you're sorry. Women could be as capricious as men, roll in Mazola oil, and do the deed with

141

whatever moved. Morals, modesty, and maternity be damned, women could act like men.

All this left out one wee scientific piece of data.

Women have a genetically driven problem with separating our bodies from our hearts. It's called oxytocin, which aids the mothering instinct to protect the replication of the species. It is a natural hormone released during sexual activity and is ramped up during the intense first six months of a relationship when there is lots 'o sex. According to author Markus McGill: "Oxytocin has an anti-anxiety (anxiolytic) effect and may increase romantic attachment and empathy. This neuropeptide exerts multiple psychological effects, influencing social behavior and emotion."

What that means in "lay" language is that once you fool around with a guy more than a handful of times you start looking for twigs to build a nest. But after those first six months of bliss the romance comes to a screeching halt and the woman finds herself screaming, "Who are you and what have you done with that nice man I married?"

News Flash: It's not him. It's the other way around. Those six months the Prince was under *your* spell...the one you cast on him with the help of oxytocin. The one where you were seeing him not only in the best possible light, but imbuing light on him that he never had a snowball's chance in hell of having. And one of the biggest projections women, as passionate sexual beings, make on this poor sucker is that he has a Lothario libido. Too often after you say the "I dos" he starts saying "I don't."

Yet sitcoms, stand-up male comics, and scientific papers tout that men want more sex and wives have "headaches." I beg to differ. In fact, I did a research study of my own, albeit with twelve women and a pitcher of Pina Coladas. Every single one admitted she wanted more sex, lots more sex, than her husband could muster up. While he plays the Demanding-Career card. She too has a demanding career, does child rearing, and housekeeping...meaning she has three freaking demanding jobs. Let's face it, you can be a sensual CEO in your cobalt business suit but when you walk through the door all your family sees is a blue chuck wagon with red lipstick on. Then your spouse asks, "What did you do all day?" ("Um, planned a funeral…yours"). Women kick butt, raise families, mourn, move on and cry so many tears we have no more left. And we still ooze passion through our size 4 or 24 jeans. Add to that we don't give a rat's ass what people think of our gray hair, wrinkles or attitude. Are we angry? You betcha. Have we been screwed over? Yeah, but only figuratively. We want respect that looks like equal pay and non-government interference with our health choices. We want to let oxytocin flow over us like purple rain and fill our hearts with love, bonding and giddiness. And that ladies is NOT too much to ask.

Now here comes the tricky part. Just when we have our act together the warranty goes out on the equipment. The aging body is a bummer. It is not just the face that goes, but the "innards" as well. Try explaining to your sweetie, who is all over you, that if he would just hold that smile and erection for fifteen minutes you'll be right back after you reattach your wig, empty your colonoscopy bag, and add some Slip-n-Slide to your nether world. Doesn't exactly conjure up Diana Krall singing, "Fly Me to The Moon."

In another study I conducted at YALE (Yolanda's All Lepkuchen Emporium), I asked my peeps to fess up. Did they want sex even with their physical pain? Yup, even with cancer, amputations, fibromyalgia, restless leg syndrome, fatigue, neuropathy, MS, and knee/hip/shoulder/liver/kidney replacements. Women can be bloated from meds, spaced out on painkillers, and vomiting from the "cures," and still want sexual touching and emotional intimacy.

Why? We are resilient. We are stronger than men. I'll stand corrected if you know of any guy who pushed an 8-pound bowling ball out of his navel…more than once. And had to potty train it. But how do you fly that sex plane with fatigued metal and a missing engine or two?

The thing is, if you love someone and they accept you the way you are, you will feel free to be you. The "new normal" or stripped down model of you means warts and all. No breasts? Scars up the yin-yang? Missing limbs? Tendency to wet the bed when cumming? Are you mortified to show, as Bridget Jones said, her wobbly bits? Here is a huge FYI. Most men don't care as long as there is a 90 percent prospect they are going to "get some." And your partner will have their issues too...heart disease, erectile no show, diabetes, and a spare tire big enough for a Monster Truck rally. All these parts come to the bedroom. Not pretty, but luckily our eyesight is going at this age.

All of your skin has nerves. Sex is the entire body not just two breasts, a vagina and a penis. It is arms, legs, fannies, necks, elbows, tongues, scalp, nape of the neck, ears, gums, inner lips, roof of mouth, shoulders, inner elbows, sides of breasts, lower back, navel, inner thighs, inner knees, toes. Sex is an exploration of mutual pleasure, not a race to the finish.

Laugh if someone farts, if your foot cramps, and yes, laugh if you fall asleep mid-sex. Smile, it's a Sunday drive with your favorite person. See where it takes you. Make-out, feel each other up, eat a banana split off each other's stomachs. Shoot whipped cream anywhere and lick it off. Sheets wash out, and who cares if they don't?

Spoiler Alert: Simultaneous orgasms are not the be-all-and-end-all. It's like having to share a birthday cake at work, not special. Take turns, it is more fun and way less stressful. Unless you enjoy faking orgasms so he thinks you came together—or was that just me? And romance does not mean silence. Who came up with the scenes in the movies where you look at each other and—wham— you just lock lips. This is a bad idea. How about asking permission and honoring a "no" answer. But if the answer is "yes," then talk about how things feel physically, what to do or stop doing. And keep talking because these things can change with every encounter! And unless you married Carnac the Magnificent, you are going to have to speak up.

If your regular receptors (read genitalia) are not in working order, it is not the end of the world. Did you know there are a bazillion places on your body that can have an orgasm? Yessiree, anywhere a bundle of nerves comes to the surface of your skin. Blam! I found this out at a boring meeting. I mindlessly started dragging a pencil eraser along the "V" shape from my thumb to my forefinger. Within three minutes my hand started to orgasm with pleasure shooting up my arm. I involuntarily moaned loudly. I have no idea what anyone said at that meeting, all I kept thinking was there must be a way to patent this little discovery of nerve bundles (hence referred to as NB). This little technique can be a godsend if traditional parts are not responding. Also during a bad movie. I just have to remember not to scream out, "Sweet-mother-of-pearl, the train is pulling into the station!"

This brings me to mutual masturbation. When starting over in romance (I am on marriage number three) you have to retrain your new Prince Charming to be, um, charming. If you were single a long time and sexual, your best friend may still be your hand-held shower massager or a plug-in device. Guess what? That can still be a part of your sexual repertoire. You do not need to be ashamed of this, bring it into your sex play together. Watch each other get off, touch their favorite NBs as they go for it. Kiss him everywhere (without getting punched in the eye by his stroking arm). Each person can get in the mood touching themselves. Then when you are both aroused you can jump on the bandwagon together.

Now, let's talk about oral sex. Take a shower first, gargle with mouthwash to kill germs that don't belong there (can you say yeast infection?) and start looking at each other's private parts like a banquet, not an embarrassment. It is even mentioned in the Bible in "The Song of Solomon": the bride sat in the groom's shadow, who is like her own apple tree, and his fruit was sweet to her taste. Then the groom puts his arm under his bride's neck and with his other hand he explores and mentions that his bride tastes like: wine, honey, pomegranates, cinnamon, saffron, and a garden fountain, to name a few.

The boudoir should be your sensual, safe, and silly space. I would heed three rules: Exhilarating not Excruciating, Bonding not Blood, and Play Nice (no passive-aggressive fallout from the day before). Make love when you have the energy, morning, noon, or during "Jeopardy." Like the old Burger King ad says, have it your way.

BRENDA YATES

DREAM SONG PHILTRE

Sometimes, after a long absence
even the long-married lie
together like strangers

stranded in an almost familiar place
where not quite understood

consonants keep tilting away
into unfamiliar language.

Sometimes even the long-married
must become more patient,

re-translate, re-interpret vowels
of hesitant mouth, tentative hand

until suddenly the old intimacies
remember desire's secret tongue

of long, sweet sex
intimate, now, and effortless.

Sometimes then, long-married
bodies, after stuttering into sleep,

curve into long slumbers of silk yesses,
yesses loud enough to waken dreams,

which, reacquainting themselves,
leave their rooms of waxy light,

and press together, talking in the low
voices of lovers, long-time lovers

who speak softly their private
dialect of hibiscus and hyacinth.

BARBARA ROCKMAN

EROTICS OF MAKING

The woman brings her body to the page
the way a climber clamps her thighs to the rock face
the way a lover drops the last garment
the way a girl crawls into a copse and, singing, arranges acorns and logs
the way a mother skips away from the departing school bus.

What is arousal?

Words at the pen tip, ink rich as clotted blood.
Hairs lifted and sinew flexed.
Grip the lid, release vinegar, cut lemon.

Row out into ooze, lean beyond the oar, raise the leg to climb over
into the silt lake bottom, toes sucked down, fear of disappearing.

Kiwi's furred cheek. Rotting peach eaten anyway. Cuticles burnt by salt.
Aged breasts relinquish what's been missed.
Blackened lilac slumped to elegy. Aretha's dropped fur.

I'm in love with women who liquefy my pen, who swing my arms out
from my sides. It happens when I enter their poem, etching, collage,
teabags hung from the spine.
One says, *After months, inspiration came.* Her face beatific, saint of the
uncensored.
One says, *In my studio, deep in the making of, I am orgasm.* She swells rice
paper into garment, each gesture a seduction.
One settles by a meadow, her soft body bent to *click click,* crow call. A
deer stares. She is so away into; she is invitation. And I am, *yes.* Without
lifting from tap and wonder, lost in dream time, she beckons. Teacher/
student? Elder/youth? No. Women.

Another's name like a razor cuts me limb from history, tugs my
fingers out and rearranges them into a new appendage. She makes
of me a placard that screams   *Violence to save the female race.* She
introduces me to her friend, Clarice.
And the long armed sister of a past life who understands addiction to
doubt   throws *Best Of* by men across the room. Pages flail like
wings of a dying breed. She takes my hands across a table scattered
with scratched out words, whispers,
We must create a new country. She works her fingers into my tangles.

These women raise a mirror, burn through glass. A marbling of
inkblots and burst meteors. When a silver surface is stripped, a black
pool gushes.
Theorist and artist, mother and lover, mentor and apprentice,
marriage bed, ocean edge: the hundred seductions, the thousand
spent bodies.
Aftermath: bliss.
I have made this; I have read you; you have listened.
We sleep the sleep of each others' dreams.
We become the tale, *Lost in the woods.* But
we return home. Purpled dusk, hour of sap.
We grip oars. We climb over the lip.

*Gratitude to Ann Laser, Cynthia Fusillo, Carole Maso, Hélène Cixous, Clarice Lispector,
and Marie Howe, mentors, friends and fellow travelers, and to all the women whose
creativity fuels my own.*

MARIANNE TAYLOR

LISTENING TO NPR DURING THE IRAQI INVASION

This voice on the radio, like raw black silk,
some Ahmad, makes me want to take off
my clothes, slip inside his sound, feel those round
vowels' assonance against my bare back--
sibilants hissing like steam on breasts and thighs--
plumb the dark warmth down his tongue with my tongue.

I pull off the highway, take in those thick vibrations
riding the airwaves like heat.
My bones are melting.
I'm oil on water in sunlight,
a gold and black puddle
pulsed with ebbing circles
on strange hot sand.

So who says
talk can't save us?

Susan Cochran

Changes

JIM WAS NOT what I was looking for. And I mean his looks. He was tall, lanky, and pale with thinning red hair and possibly wearing polyester pants and shirt, if I remember correctly. We hardly spoke the same language—he was a software engineer with a physics and computer background and I was an English major in my junior year of college. But there was this attraction, this feeling that when he looked at me, he saw the real me. There was a sense of calmness in our meeting. No great seduction, no overt flirting, just an awareness of where we were in a crowded room.

It was spring 1979 and I had volunteered to pour wine at the La Jolla Ski Club's Spring Dance. I was twenty-seven at the time and just coming out of a divorce. I'd married young, caught up in the happily-ever-after dream, but we grew up and away from each other. Single for the first time since eighteen, I'd started dating but wasn't making the connections that were important to me.

I danced with Jim and other men that evening. Jim walked me to my car and he kissed me, again and again under the streetlight on a warm San Diego night. I drove home knowing he would call to set up that date like he said he would. The next day, I got several calls from a bored on-duty fireman I met at that same dance. No fires meant calling me but he wasn't the one I wanted to talk to. I unplugged my phone and went for a walk through Balboa Park, knowing that Jim would eventually call; I didn't have to wait around.

We took it slow: a sailing date the next weekend, dinners out, walks and long talks for the next month. More kissing and caressing but we didn't seem to be in a hurry for more. Then we both went on a Salt River Rafting trip out of Phoenix with the ski club. I'd already set up to room with a girlfriend and Jim was rooming with a guy friend. That first day was spent at the pool and dancing that evening. We were obviously a couple but went off to our respective rooms late that night. The next day was the raft trip and we laughed and splashed our way down the river and more dancing that night. My roommate approached me and said she'd already talked with Jim's roommate and they could room together so Jim and I could spend the night together. I thanked her but said it wasn't necessary. I didn't want to be the talk of the club and I felt that we'd have more chances to get together, not one manufactured by others. It didn't have to happen then or not at all. Jim took it in stride and this opened the conversation about deepening our relationship when it was right for us. We sat curled together on the long bus ride back to San Diego.

The time we put into getting to know and understand each other seemed to strengthen our attraction. We laughed about it afterward, but we were both worried that sex would complicate this relationship we'd built. Instead it brought a new closeness. Both coming out of divorces, we were in awe that we found such a new depth to love. It was a healing time for us, too, our previous marriage experiences had left us wounded and doubtful of finding someone we could trust.

I remember that before Jim, I always did what was "right" and worked hard to meet others' expectations of being "a good girl," and the results weren't pretty. So I simply went with my intuition and heart, and knew there was a comfort, a security, a deep connection with Jim. We moved in together that summer. When we wrote our wedding vows in December that year, we intentionally left out "until death do us part" because we knew that everything changes. And, ironically, that is exactly what separated us.

So. This brings us to the "sex after fifty" part of this essay. Jim and I were married for thirty years. Sex during that time was what I would think most women have in a long-term monogamous relationship: thrilling, amazing, routine, one more thing to do on the list, no, no again, yes, yes again, baby-making-sex, pregnancy sex, sex when the kids are asleep, sex when the kids are out of the house, sex in different rooms/beds/cities/countries, and the last several years of the marriage (here is the after fifty part) I found sex to be a comforting closeness and sensual familiarity as both our bodies were changing with age and we were adapting together.

He was my home.

On the Fourth of July, 2010, Jim had a fatal heart attack on a bike ride. No warning. Just an abrupt end to a world that was so familiar. I was plunged into an ocean of grief; sometimes drowning, sometimes treading water, sometimes drifting and then being dragged below by an undertow of sorrow. That first year was tumultuous with the grieving and the business of being a widow. I filled out form after form, but the full impact came when I met with my tax person. I asked where the box was for "widowed," because the only other choices were married or single. So, like a flip of a switch, I understood that I was single. Again.

Coupling was the last thing on my mind. In fact, with my Plan A taken away, I needed to give myself time to find my Plan B. I was well versed in *us* and I wanted to know what just me would be like. There have been still more changes as I get a handle on this single thing. I try not to idealize Jim and laugh that we were the perfect imperfect. The quandary of what makes me happy has been a great adventure. I've made mistakes and had successes. I've had to let go of my opinions as I wander into the land of the unfettered and bounce between independence and profound loneliness. Desire is just below the surface at times, like a ripple from the past and an anticipation of the future.

Passion has expanded its meaning for me. Travel opportunities were presented soon after his death and I've come to love planning to visit a new country and the experiences it brings. Jim always made the travel arrangements and I was the companion and sometimes whiner when things didn't go right. I was worried I wouldn't travel again after losing Jim. But an invitation came from old friends to help with their olive harvest in Cortona, Italy, that October. I said yes and then had to get myself there. I made the arrangements and the date of travel landed on what would have been Jim's sixtieth birthday. The middle seat on the flight from LAX to Rome was empty and upon waking from dozing, I imagined Jim's presence traveling with me. How appropriate there was room for him.

The physical work of harvesting olives was demanding and the camaraderie of new and old friends a comfort. My room overlooked a beautiful countryside and, missing Jim one morning, I cried as the sun came up over the trees. The yearning for the past and fear of a future without him was such a part of my present. Then I had to laugh that he would hate the work of a harvest, this would not have been his idea of a vacation. I would have to come up with my own ideas. And this one worked.

The first anniversary of his death, I was on a walking tour of the Wye Valley in Wales. The travel dates were happenstance and fell over the Fourth of July. It was great to be in a country where that holiday was of no matter. A friend woke me on that morning and said there was a cup of tea and a biscuit for me on the table and I should come down to breakfast after I've made peace with the morning. Later that day, as the hiking group made their way down the trail, I sat alone on the hill. Blue skies, white marshmallow clouds, patchwork quilt fields and the river snaking its long winding way through the valley was before me. How could all not be right with the world on a day such as this? I realized that I may not like what happened, but I had to learn how to live with it.

It has been six years since Jim died and so much has changed. At times I feel I am an observer of life. I watch couples as they go about their normal lives and marvel at my single friends who live a fulfilled life. Time does not stop and grieve. The hours, days and months tick on and I've had to adapt. I've sensed a new way to look at couples as idealized in our society and a new bravery to feel whole, just as I am.

Some of my friends and family are curious as to why I haven't ordered another man. Or at least this is what online dating seems to me. Advertise myself and click on one of them. If my friends know single women who have "found a man" they get the details to tell me so I will know how it was done. Someone told me not to worry, that there was still time. Or friends will point to guys and say *how about him* or *him over there?* Apparently expecting me to go up and say brightly, "I'm available." I've also been accused of not looking. Walking with a friend at the beach, she pointed out that a guy said hi as he walked by and I ignored him. And it was true; I wasn't looking.

It is not that I haven't thought about being with a man. I miss the love, tenderness, intimacy, and physical connection. I also miss the history with Jim. I will carry that history to the next man and he will bring his history to me.

So. I've looked into dating and it has changed. When I last dated, I was worried about getting pregnant. Now safe sex is at the forefront of new relationships no matter how old you are. At my last checkup, my doctor asked me if there was anything I wanted to discuss. I said I was contemplating dating after thirty years in a monogamous relationship. Anything new? She pulled up a chair and I got the full report on being sexually active at my age and what I or my partner may bring to the bed...so to speak.

So. I'm still working on the man thing. I met a very nice man but it was obvious I wanted more than just sex and it seemed to be difficult for him to spend the time getting to know me. There is also a fear of a man consuming my life. I'm a committer and I wonder how I would fit a man into my active life.

I have a great many wonderful friends. Retired now, I play tennis and hike and bike with different groups. I train with a team for the summer sprint triathlon. These activities provide a physical outlet as well as being out in nature. I take classes at the local community college in creative writing and photography. I see so many details of beauty through the lens of the camera Jim held in his hands, and writing can take me to places that are untouched. I love the ocean and have spent many hours on the beach watching the tides turn and realizing the cycles of my life are an ebb and flow of history and experience and things to come—most times out of my control—but my inner self can be the peaceful point on that compass of my life. I still travel quite a bit and I've been out of the country every Fourth of July since Jim's death. A sort of pilgrimage to center myself in an unknown place and realize that life has so much to offer if I put myself out there.

I won't let traveling as a single stop me. I once sat next to a young woman at Charles De Gaulle Airport in Paris. As we talked, she explained she was going to spend a week in Rome with an aunt and uncle. She apologetically explained that she was traveling alone and her relatives worked so she'd be sadly seeing the sights by herself. I said that due to circumstances, I was on my way to Spain for three weeks traveling alone. I laughingly said we could be home sitting on couches waiting for someone to come and save us, but instead we get to visit new and exciting countries in Europe. I stressed it is just as valuable if we're on own. Drink in all the museums and architecture and winding walks and people and it will fill the imagination.

It is a good, unexpected life, and I am so lucky to have such a solid past to build upon. I try to keep a positive attitude and an expectancy of great things to come. I'm open to share it with that special man, but before that happens I'm not going to miss a thing. I may even start "clicking," and I actually said "hi" to a man on the street today. I noticed.

MINDELA RUBY

MAQUILLAGE

In putting on makeup
Definition is the goal
You add it
These ways:
Outline
Color
Darken
Lighten
Erase

Pick a look or fashion
Your mood to convey
Decide whether to apply
Any makeup at all

I never took
Cosmetics seriously
Even with daily daubs
But age requires
The art of
Maquillage
If one doesn't want
To look a fright
Which is why
I learned to shape
The contours of
A lived-in face:
Omit old shadows
Paint new angles

Blot out spots
Make my kisser bright

I work my face
I reinvent it
I put on more makeup
And go to bed

Maria Keane

Aging in Winter

Frost
scores my window.
Linear explorations,
abstract etchings cluster.
They burst forth in
cracklings and
give no hint
of direction: lines
that weather years. But then,
your compassionate breath
heats the surface of my wintering
to melt
my map of aging
into liquid, washing years away.

Renata Golden

Frank's Daughters

I HAD BEEN INTRIGUED by his photo on the online dating site for almost two years. The hip goatee, the sweater draped over his shoulders, the thoughtful, sanguine face and the charming smile. In one photograph, he wore a beret pulled down over his forehead with a flair that worked perfectly for a retired architect. At six-foot-five and slender, he carried his sixty-five years with grace.

His age made me uncomfortable, but I reasoned that a seven-year difference wasn't a deal breaker in the larger scheme of things. More important, I was encouraged by something he had written. "What are we valuing, thinking, saying? Is it kind, generous, fun?" A cut above the "Renaissance man/Harley biker looking for a classy lady" types. The other men on the site clearly specified what they wanted and what they didn't. A camping/fishing/skiing buddy half their age. No games, no baggage, no cats. My architect wrote, "We are all here together hanging onto this spinning ball so...passionate about love and connection."

In those two years on Match, I endured a succession of libido-numbing first dates. Over each coffee, lunch, and dinner, I hoped to step into the heart of my next life partner, or at least onto the calendar of a kindred spirit. But after kissing goodbye to a pond-full of frogs, I tried not to lose heart. Although eager for success, I wanted to take my time before getting involved, to savor the moments of discovery and delight and even distaste. But first I needed to meet someone worth a second date.

Being cautious was something I learned at a young age from my father, Lt. Frank Golden, a cop on the South Side of Chicago. He had strict rules for his three daughters, especially concerning safety, especially around men. Don't open the door if you don't know who's on the other side, don't accept rides from strangers, don't trust anyone you don't know. And don't believe everything you hear. My father's voice echoed as I searched the architect's profile; he would have been appalled by the concept of online dating. I had decided to end my subscription to the service, but first I sent one more message.

"Every time I stumble across your profile, I see someone I would like to get to know," I wrote. "However, I'm quitting Match. I emailed you once before but never heard back, which I should take as an indication of your interest. I am trying again, though, because I won't ever know if I don't try, right?"

The next morning a message waited in my inbox. "I was/am attracted, but busy ending a long-distance affair. I'm not so good at that or at communicating with two women at once...am old-fashioned, I think. So I must end one before starting up new. But much thanks. Frank."

It wasn't a total rejection, although the long distance made me nervous. He lived in the California Bay Area; I lived in the Southwest. Where did the woman he was breaking up with live? I reread the sentence "I was/am attracted." I renewed my subscription.

The slippery, frustrating, frightening elusiveness of a connection made me question everything I thought I knew about relationships and my ability to have one. I launched a give-a-frog-a-chance campaign, in the off chance that my ability to recognize a prince-in-waiting was impaired. The net result was I wasted a lot of time and sent a lot of great-to-meet-you-but messages.

I kept faith that the ingredients for connection hadn't gone extinct. My father had taught me everything he knew about kindness and compassion. Ironically, as a lawman, his knowledge in that department was significant. He was also a role model for a happy marriage; my parents had taken their vows until death seriously. I took it as a good sign that he and my architect shared the same name.

Six months later, when I needed to be in California for business, I emailed Frank to ask about getting together. He responded immediately and in all caps. "YES!"

"Let's stay in touch," he wrote. "I am recovering from a cold...it's all that's kept me from heading your way. Would be nice to meet... am sure we share much."

I didn't have a checklist, but if I did, he would have met it. Tall and handsome, check. Articulate and artistic, check. He was clear about what he was looking for in a partner. "She will be compassionate and understanding...affectionate and loving (need that be said?)" His best line: "Intimacy makes the ordinary extraordinary...like sleeping (ya know, when I put my arm around her and her leg slides in between mine)."

"I have dates for my visit," I emailed. "Will you be around the middle of next month?"

He responded that he was traveling but would be home soon. "Rented a house at Donner Lake. Backpacked with my son to find places to take the grandchildren this winter. Want to teach them how to ski."

"I'm in meetings on Monday, but am flexible after that. How's your schedule?"

"Leaving Tuesday and Wednesday open...for you. Anything together could be fun. See you soonish."

I imagined meeting this man, flirting with someone who towered over me. I pictured myself laughing at his jokes, leaning into him to feel his heat. I felt more optimistic—and less suspicious—than I had felt in years.

"I'm here in Fremont," I wrote on Sunday when I arrived. "I hope you had a good weekend."

"Well, Serena won, the 49ers won, and the Giants won...but it was only because of my cold that I stayed in and watched."

"Will we still be able to get together?" I wrote back.

"Are we on for Tuesday or Wednesday? Had some intensive acupuncture treatments last week, did I tell you? Another one planned for tomorrow. It takes time to process, so Wednesday is better, if that works for you. I'll know tomorrow. Alas, the treatment is highest priority since standard medicine didn't help. Will call ASAP."

Wednesday felt like a long time to wait to finally hear his voice. I shut down my laptop and went to bed early, anticipating a full workday. When my cell phone rang at 11 p.m., I remembered my father's dictum growing up—no one worth talking to calls after 10. I never considered Frank would call so late. When he called again at 9 Monday morning, this time he left a message.

"Are you really there? Do you ever pick up your phone? Let's talk about this week. Call me." I was beguiled by his voice—sexy, deep, and calm. I replayed the message three times before setting my phone to vibrate.

At the first break in my meeting, I called his cell phone and left a message. "I turned my phone off, but I'm checking email."

"It's hard for me to talk after an acupuncture treatment," he wrote that evening. "But I expect to feel fine tomorrow. We can talk around 10. And you can email me anytime."

Tuesday morning 10 came and went. When I checked my email about an hour later, there was a note from Frank. "I can pick you up today wherever you are staying. We can have lunch or dinner in Berkeley or San Francisco. Let me know what works for you."

"I can't get away for lunch, but dinner in Berkeley sounds great," I emailed. I was surprised and delighted he decided not to wait until Wednesday. "I can meet you. Just let me know where and when."

"Do you like Italian? I know a place in my neighborhood. If BART works for you, there is a train station about four blocks from the restaurant. I can pick you up there. Is a 6:30 or 7:30 reservation okay?"

When I had a break around noon, I left another message on his cell phone. "I can be in Berkeley by 6:30. What time is the reservation?"

My meetings ended at 3:30, but I hadn't heard from Frank. Was he having second thoughts? I pushed aside my doubts and sent him another email, and then returned to my hotel to dress for dinner. When Frank hadn't called me by 4:30 I called him again—this time on his home number.

"Hi, Frank, it's me," I said.

"Hello," a woman's voice responded. My heart skipped a beat. "This is Frank's daughter." Then she hesitated. "I'm really sorry to tell you this, but my father passed away today."

His daughter continued to talk but I'm not really sure what she said. I was wondering why she was the one saying she was sorry when she just lost her father. I was wondering why she didn't sound more distraught. Had she known this was coming? I was picturing Frank's face in that photograph I looked at so often—that smile, those eyes. I couldn't believe that his picture was all I would ever have.

"I'm so sorry," I said, wondering how many times I had emailed or called a dead man.

"Can I ask how you knew my father?" she asked.

This time I hesitated. Should I tell her we had been communicating online? Should I tell her we never met—had never even spoken to each other? "We were supposed to have dinner tonight," I stammered.

"Oh, Renata." She said my name as if she had known me forever. "He told me he had a date with you tonight. I'm so sorry."

What exactly did Frank tell her and when? Was the last conversation Frank had about me? My grief felt selfish and misplaced. What was appropriate to say to Frank's daughter? It seemed that all we could do was trade apologies. "I'm so sorry. Can I ask what happened?"

"I really don't know. He looks peaceful. He's just sitting in his chair."

I recalled the headline Frank had written on his dating profile. "If this were the last day of our lives, what would we be doing together?" I now knew the answer, but it was all wrong. We wouldn't be doing anything together, not today, not any day. His question, and all of mine, hung in the air.

I had Googled Frank; I knew he lived in Berkeley and had been an architect. But now, starved for a connection, I dug deeper. A personal information website showed a little plus sign after his age: sixty-five-plus. I assumed that meant he was sixty-five years old plus some ever-increasing months. But the internet told me he was irrefutably seventy-six. How did he expect to hide that from me? Who had I agreed to get into a car with at the BART stop? For two weeks I searched obituaries in the Bay Area but never found a listing for him. It didn't matter—the Frank I thought I knew was dead.

Some fathers teach their daughters how to save themselves needless pain. And some fathers teach their daughters that pain can be a tool. That is, if the woman who answered the phone when I called Frank's house was really his daughter. And if he had really died. Her use of present tense—"He looks peaceful. He's just sitting in his chair."—haunted me. Was she really looking at her dead father? Or was she looking at a man trying to get out of a blind date?

The survival skills my father taught me were designed to protect me as a woman in the world. They were skills I had been in danger of forgetting. My father was married to my mother for forty years, until first she, then he, died. A forty-year marriage is something I will never have. In its place I have advice from a father to his daughter and a passion for love and connection. I also have a newly learned lesson about the difficulties of ending my search. I renewed my subscription to the dating service, fully aware that I was opening a door without knowing who was on the other side.

CATHLEEN CALBERT

FLOWER-EATING SEASON

It's spring, and my dazed dog
        devours all flowers, our walks
                punctuated by munches. She's more
        than happy, gulping down small blue flutes
and decapitating dandelions,
        a flower-glutton of a mutt, and so I think
                of cunnilingus, what a struggle
        for some men to get down on their knees,
that boy a thousand years ago
        who said *I like it*
                because you like it,
        which made me never want him
to push his face between my legs again,
        though you, husband, used to assiduously
                put your mouth upon my flower
        when we were young(ish) and green(ery)
until I newly bloomed, shall we say.
        What's taking her so long?
                asked one young man watching
        a "sex awareness" film as the woman
on screen swam twenty minutes
        toward the shore of her orgasm,
                those slow sweet strokes far
        from porn or whores or this old guy,
"friend of the family," whose "supported,
        sorta" girlfriend, one third his age, comes,
                he tells me, three times in ten minutes.
        No, she doesn't, I want to say.
Are you an idiot? I want to say
        to my husband. *It's flower-eating season.*

167

What lies before us but aging and death?
Remember how we slept
in the same big bed and you weren't
too fatigued to please me? Instead
I walk my crazy girl, who wants to
swallow the world, and I've bought myself
a vase full of flowers: red roses surrounded
by irises and orchids as wild as pink leopards.
Well, there's always my own hand
and still your kind smile. I'm faithful,
or at least not unfaithful, as Larkin
might have said, though I must say
I turn these days more to Cummings.

JULIE WENGLINSKI

ONE MORE MORNING

Beneath a mostly cloudy sky
I unearth myself
from a tangle of cats and faded quilts
sit up
and with slow half focus
reconnect with my conscious self.
I take a small and yellow pill
and wait for the anxious to pass.
With half scrubbed face,
fan of bed smashed hair,
and sequinned slippers,
I step downstairs in the unraveling blue kimono,
to join you on the glider
where you swing softly with your coffee,
next to the checkered woodpeckers.
And I, with blurred morning vision,
see your blue eyes taking me in,
and my own reflection in your shine.
I tuck the solid soundness of you within my chest
where the anxious was.

ACKNOWLEDGMENTS

"Orgasmic Harley, or Where Are My Balls," (Bernadette Murphy) is excerpted from *Harley and Me, Embracing Risk on the Road to a More Authentic Life*, Counterpoint Press, 2016.

"The Widow Revives," (Phyllis Wax) originally appeared under a slightly different title in *The Widow's Handbook, Poetic Reflections on Grief and Survival*, Kent State University Press.

"I Chose an Eastern King," (Lori White) first appeared at *The Nervous Breakdown* (thenervousbreakdown.com) in January 2015.

"In the Museum of Fucking," (Louise Marie Harrod) originally appeared in *Poems & Plays*.

"Two Worlds," (Diane Raab) from *Lust*, CW Books, 2014.

"Unrepentant Body," (Becky Dennison Sakellariou) appeared in *Persimmon Tree* in 2010 and in *The Possibility of Red*, a bilingual chapbook (Greek and English), in 2013.

"Philomon and Baucis," (Eva Haller) originally appeared in Thrive online.

"Anniversary," (Davi Walders) previously appeared in *A More Perfect Union* (St. Martin's Press) and has been read by Garrison Keillor on The Writer's Almanac.

"Sex on the Sand," (Irene Fick) was originally published in *Gargoyle Magazine*, February 2016.

Editors

Marcia Meier is an award-winning writer, editor, and publisher of Weeping Willow Books. Her work has appeared in *The Louisville Review*, Writersresist.com, *Prime Number Magazine* online, the anthology *Knocking at the Door, Approaching the Other*, the *Los Angeles Times*, Huffington Post, and many other publications. Her books include *Ireland, Place Out of Time* (2017); *Heart on a Fence* (2016); *Navigating the Rough Waters of Today's Publishing World, Critical Advice for Writers from Industry Insiders* (2010); and *Santa Barbara, Paradise on the Pacific* (1996). She is at work on a memoir.

Kathleen A. Barry, Ph.D., has been a licensed psychotherapist in California since 1995 and specializes in working with individuals as they face the crossroads of major life transitions. She has published a variety of writings about women, empowerment, grief, and sexuality on her website: www.whispersofwisdom.com.

Dr. Barry is an adjunct professor at Antioch University, Santa Barbara, where she teaches a variety of courses in the bachelor of arts program.

CONTRIBUTORS

RIRA ABBASI is an Iranian poet, fiction writer and peace activist. Acclaimed as Iran's Lady Poet Laureate and the winner of the Parvin Etesami Poetry Award in 2005, Rira is also a member of Iran's Writers Association and the founder and director of the biennial International Peace Poetry Festival since 2007. *Black Fairy of Wednesday* (2000), *No More Guns for This Lor Woman* (2001) and a bold collection of love poems, *Who Loves You More Discreetly?* (2002) are among her works. Rira has edited and introduced the first collection of Iranian Peace Poetry (an anthology) in 2002. A brainchild of Rira Abbasi and supported solely by individual donations and sponsorship of non-governmental organizations, the charter of the Peace Poetry Festival states that "Poetry for peace is affiliated to humanity, regardless of race, religion, sex and geography."

MARYAM ALA AMJADI is an Iranian poet, essayist, and translator who spent the impressionable years of her childhood in India and writes poetry in English. She is the author of two poetry collections and translator of a collection of Raymond Carver's poems into Farsi. She received the Young Generation Poet Award in the first International Poetry Festival in Yinchuan, China (Sept 2011) and was awarded Honorary Fellowship in Creative Writing by the International Writers Program (IWP) at the University of Iowa in fall 2008. She is a Ph.D. research fellow in Text and Event in Early Modern Europe (TEEME) at the universities of Kent (UK) and Porto (Portugal). She is also an editor for *Hysteria*, a periodical of critical feminisms. Her poems have been translated into Arabic, Albanian, Chinese, Hindi, Italian and Romanian.

BAMBI BARKER is a pen name for an established poet. Bambi has published poetry in *A Kiss is Still a Kiss* from Outrider Press, *Shoes Magazine*, *Poetry Greece*, *Cokefishing*, *The Diddler*, *Love's Chance*, *Poems Niederngasse* (Switzerland), *Mannequin Envy*, *Lummox*, *Nefarious Ballerina*, *Zen Baby*, *Zygote in My Coffee*, *The Centrifugal Eye*, *Sein und Werden* (England), and *The Scribbler*. She has read her poetry on the LUVER radio station, has worked as a model for a foot fetish website, and is way over fifty years old.

CATHARINE BRAMKAMP publishes both prose and poetry. Her poetry has been included in a dozen anthologies, including *And The Beats Go On* (which she edited) and the chapbook *Ammonia Sunrise* (Finishing Line Press). She is co-producer of the Newbie Writers Podcast and teaches at two universities. She has written fourteen novels and three books on writing. She is the chief storytelling officer for three companies, because social media can be a lot like poetry.

DEBBIE BROSTEN relocated to Bellingham, WA, after retiring from a career in education. She delights in the serendipity of her travel-filled life and the people who populate it. Her work has been published in the *Whatcom Writes Anthology; Memory into Memoir: A Red Wheelbarrow Writers Collection;* and *Give Yourself Permission Anthology.*

RITA BULLINGER, a blue belle in a red zone, is a writer and feminist living in the southern United States. She has written for small publications in the San Francisco Bay Area and in the southeast, and writes a blog called "Out of the Blue" about literature, politics, and the natural world, including sex.

CAROLYN BUTCHER, PH.D., teaches critical thinking through literature at Santa Barbara City College in California. Her memoir work has appeared in several online and print journals, most recently in *Spring: A Journal of Archetype and Culture*, and for many years she presented academic papers at James Joyce conferences internationally. In addition, she has read her personal essays at several performances of *Speaking of Stories* at Center Stage Theater in Santa Barbara. She is grateful to her husband, Michael Dean Perry, her two children, two grandchildren, and two stepchildren for all their love and support.

CATHLEEN CALBERT's poetry and prose have appeared in many publications, including *Ms. Magazine, The New Republic, The New York Times,* and *The Paris Review.* She is the author of four books of poetry: *Lessons in Space, Bad Judgment, Sleeping with a Famous Poet,* and *The Afflicted Girls.* Her awards include The Nation Discovery Award, a Pushcart Prize, the Sheila Motton Book Prize, the Vernice Quebodeaux Poetry Prize for Women, and the Mary Tucker Thorp Award from Rhode Island College.

SUSAN COCHRAN grew up in the San Fernando Valley and earned a B.A. in English from San Diego State University and an English Teaching Credential from San Jose State University. While working in administration at the University of California, Santa Barbara, Susan expressed her creativity through quilt art and painting. After the death of her husband, she turned to journaling and poetry. She received the first place prize for the 2013 Robert J. Emmons Poetry Competition and completed the Creative Writing Certificate Program at Santa Barbara City College. Her short memoir story, *Aztec Street*, was published in *Thoreau's Rooster,* Assumption College. Her poetry has been used at Hospice of Santa Barbara to help the healing of loss. Her recently published book, *In the Sea of Grief and Love*, shares her experiences with grief.

PAM DAVENPORT settled in the Sonoran Desert after traveling the world throughout her childhood. She has an MFA from Pacific University and her poems have recently appeared in *The Avalon Literary Review, Snapdragon, Rougarou, Pittsburgh Poetry Review, Spilled Milk Magazine,* and *Bared: An Anthology on Bras and Breasts.*

Lisa del Rosso originally trained as a classical singer and completed a post-graduate program at the London Academy of Music and Dramatic Art, living and performing in London before moving to New York City. Her plays "Clare's Room," and "Samaritan," have been performed off-Broadway and had public readings, while "St. John," her third play, was a semi-finalist for the 2011 Eugene O'Neill National Playwrights Conference. Her writing has appeared in *The New York Times, Barking Sycamores Neurodivergent Literature, Razor's Edge Literary Magazine, The Literary Traveler, Serving House Journal, VietnamWarPoetry, Young Minds Magazine* (London/UK), *Time Out New York, The Huffington Post, The Neue Rundschau* (Germany), *Jetlag Café* (Germany), and *One Magazine* (London/UK), for whom she writes theater reviews. She teaches writing at NYU.

Lisa Mae DeMasi's work has been featured in the literary journals *Vine Leaves* (May 2017), *Gravel, Slippery Elm, Foliate Oak, East Bay Review, Shark Reef,* and several media outlets including HuffPost. When she's not writing, she practices Reiki, specializing in unblocking creatives in all mediums and moving them (with humor and love) to the highest vision of themselves as artists.

Liz Rose Dolan's poetry manuscript, *A Secret of Long Life,* nominated for the Robert McGovern Prize, has been published by Cave Moon Press. Her first collection, *They Abide,* was published by March Street. A nine-time Pushcart nominee and winner of Best of the Web, she was a finalist for Best of the Net 2014.

Haiden Fairly is a senior administrator for a non-profit organization in Santa Barbara. She loves being out in nature, biking, hiking or watching birds. Her creative passions in life are writing and acting. She has been married to the same man for thirty-seven years, they have two adult children, and they still have sex together.

ALEXIS RHONE FANCHER is the author of *How I Lost My Virginity To Michael Cohen and Other Heart Stab Poems*, and *State of Grace: The Joshua Elegies*. Her erotic poems have been featured in more than sixty journals and lit magazines, including *Little Raven, Cactus Heart, Red Light Lit, Slipstream, Cliterature, Cleaver, Menacing Hedge, Rattle, Hobart, Broadzine*, and *Gutter Eloquence*. Since 2013 Alexis has been nominated for seven Pushcart Prizes and four Best of The Net awards. She's infamous for her Lit Crawl LA performances at Romantix, a NoHo sex shop. In her other life, Alexis is poetry editor of *Cultural Weekly*, where she also publishes a monthly photo essay, *The Poet's Eye*. alexisrhonefancher.com

ROBERTA FEINS received her MFA in poetry in 2007 from New England College. Her poems have been published in *Five AM, Antioch Review, The Cortland Review*, and *The Gettysburg Review*, among others. Her chapbook *Something Like a River*, was published by Moon Path Press in 2013. Roberta edits the e-zine *Switched On Gutenberg* (www.switched-ongutenberg.org)

IRENE FICK'S first collection of poetry, *The Stories We Tell*, was published in 2014 by The Broadkill Press. The book received first place awards (book of verse) from the National Federation of Press Women (NFPW) and the Delaware Press Association (DPA). Irene's poetry has been published in such journals as *Poet Lore; Gargoyle; The Broadkill Review; Philadelphia Stories; Adanna Literary Journal; Mojave River Review;* and *Delaware Beach Life*. Her poetry has been nominated for a Pushcart Prize. In 2016, Irene's poem, "Asunder," received the first place award from DPA, and second place from NFPW. She lives in Lewes, DE, with her husband.

LOLA FONTAY lives on the Pacific Ocean in Southern California. She is a writer and a lover of cats and men of all ages.

ANGELA M. FRANKLIN is a poet, essayist, and visual artist. She is a 2016 Fellow for the Community Literature Initiative, a 2015 Fellow for the Nora Zeale Hurston/Richard Wright Summer Writers Workshop, and a 2015 Fellow for the Voices of Our Nation Art (VONA) of Southern California. Franklin's first book of poetry, *Poems Beneath My Keloids*, is forthcoming from World Stage Press in 2018. Her poetry debuted in *Leimert Park Redux*, an anthology, and in Cultural Weekly. As a fervent supporter of impoverished women and children, she uses her energies to support efforts and causes to lift them out of poverty through clean water and education projects. She is a regular participant of the Poetry of Social Justice Workshop in Los Angeles, where she joins diverse poets to offer reflections and responses in verse on social issues and challenges.

SALLY FRANZ is a published author with multiple awards from The Santa Barbara Writers Conference. Her published work includes: "Monster Lies" a co-authored non-fiction work by Beagle Bay Books. Also, *The Baby Boomers Mini-Field Guides*, a three-book series consisting of guides to: "Menopause, Raising Teenagers, and Co-dependency" as well as "I Love You When." All humor books published by Nightingale Press, UK. Anthology contributions include the *New York Times* Best Selling: *Chicken Soup for the Grandparent's Soul*. She is a contributing blogger to *The Third Age* e-magazine. She has been a national speaker appearing on "The Today Show" three times, "The Maury Povitch Show" and "Lifetime" cable. She lives with her innkeeper husband, Dwight, in the Pacific Northwest, on the Olympic Peninsula next to Olympic National Park.

MAYA SHAW GALE, M.A. is a poet, playwright and performance artist with a passion for combining movement and the spoken word. She has performed in Santa Barbara for Poetry Month, Santa Barbara ADAPT Festival and Nectar, in Santa Barbara Bolero with Larry Kegwin and Co, and staged readings of her play, "They Say She Is Veiled," and "Five Foot Feat," a dance and disability theater piece that toured California and New York City. Her first book of poetry, *The Last Wild Place* was published in 2011, and more than twenty of her poems have appeared in two books of collected works, *The Pepper Lane Review, I* and *II*. Maya is also a transformational life coach, integrating mindfulness, wisdom from Nature and a body-centered approach to guide clients through transition to a more authentic and soul-nourishing lifestyle. She also leads dream workshops and women's writing retreats called Write From the Heart.

Renata Golden holds an MFA in creative writing from the University of Houston. She runs a technical writing company and has been an instructor at the Institute of American Indian Arts in Santa Fe, NM. In addition to having published several textbooks by HPE Press, Renata has been published in *Terrain.org* as well as newspapers across the country. Originally from the South Side of Chicago, Renata lives in Santa Fe and is working on an essay collection about the Chiricahua Mountains.

Ana Garza G'z has an MFA from California State University, Fresno. Over sixty of her poems have appeared in various journals and anthologies, most recently in *Breath and Shadow*. She works as a lecturer, community interpreter, and translator.

Eva Haller is a much-honored nonprofit leader and philanthropist. For the past three decades, she and her husband, Dr. Yoel Haller, have been devoted to social, educational and environmental activism. Earlier in her life, she was co-founder of the Campaign Communications Institute of America, a highly successful consulting firm that revolutionized the use of telephone marketing by Fortune 100 companies and political campaigns. For more than seventeen years, she served as board chair of Free the Children USA (now part of WE Charity)—which partners with communities to work from within to break the cycle of poverty. She is a trustee of the Rubin Museum of Art and the University of California Santa Barbara Foundation and serves on the boards of the Creative Visions Foundation, Sing for Hope, Video Volunteers, Asia Initiatives, and A Blade of Grass. In 2015, she was appointed to the Advisory of the Prince's Charities, the Canadian charitable office of HRH the Prince of Wales.

Lois Marie Harrod's sixteenth and most recent collection, *Nightmares of the Minor Poet*, appeared in June 2016 from Five Oaks. Her chapbook *And She Took the Heart* appeared in January 2016, and *Fragments from the Biography of Nemesis* (Cherry Grove Press) and the chapbook *How Marlene Mae Longs for Truth* (Dancing Girl Press) appeared in 2013. *The Only Is* won the 2012 Tennessee Chapbook Contest (Poems & Plays), and *Brief Term*, a collection of poems about teachers and teaching was published by Black Buzzard Press, 2011. *Cosmogony* won the 2010 Hazel Lipa Chapbook (Iowa State). She is widely published in literary journals and online ezines from *American Poetry Review* to *Zone 3*. She teaches Creative Writing at The College of New Jersey. loismarieharrod.org.

Tanya (Hyonhye) Ko Hong, poet, translator and cultural curator has been published in *Rattle, Beloit Poetry Journal, Two Hawks Quarterly, Portside, Cultural Weekly, Korea Times, Korea Central Daily News* and elsewhere. She has an MFA in creative writing from Antioch University in Los Angeles, and is the author of four books of poetry, most recently, *Mother to Myself, A collection of poems in Korean* (Prunsasang Press, 2015). Her poem, "Comfort Woman" won honorable mention in the 2015 Women's National Book Association awards. She created the reading, "Bittersweet: The Immigrant Stories," which was a Poets & Writers-sponsored reading and workshop. Tanya is an advocate of bilingual poetry, promoting the work of immigrant poets. She lives in Palos Verdes, CA, where she makes a killer oxtail soup and dances every Monday at six o'clock. tanyakohong.com

Maria Keane is an award-winning artist and published poet. She served as an adjunct professor of fine arts at Wilmington University from 1984-2008. Maria is an Arts and Letters member of the National League of American Pen Women. Her prints, paintings and poetry have received awards of excellence in national and local exhibitions. Maria is a juried member of the National Association of Women Artists (NYC), a signature member of the Philadelphia Water Color Society, and a member of the Howard Pyle Studio Group in Wilmington, DE. She has contributed to poetry collections celebrating art at the Biggs Museum of American Art from 2005-2011. In 1997, Maria received a Professional Fellowship in Works on Paper, jointly endowed by the NEA and the Delaware Division of the Arts.

DIANE KIMBALL has read and composed poems since the age of ten. She has been an educator for nearly fifty years, and retired from teaching languages and history in the public schools to write. Diane has published essays and poems in *The Bear River Review*, *The Crazy Wisdom Community Journal* and other current events periodicals. She teaches yoga and creative writing to her fellow seniors in Hilo, Hawai'i. She is at work on a family memoir titled *Across the Ponds*. Diane returns to her home state of Michigan in the summer to explore what *place* really means in one's life.

JENNIFER LAGIER, sixty-seven, has published twelve books and in literary magazines, taught with California Poets in the Schools, co-edits the *Homestead Review*, and helps coordinate Monterey Bay Poetry Consortium Second Sunday readings. Newest books: *Scene of the Crime* (Evening Street Press) and *Harbingers* (Blue Light Press). Forthcoming chapbook: *Camille Abroad* (FutureCycle). jlagier.net

SUSAN LANDGRAF is the author of the poetry collection, *What We Bury Changes the Ground*, published by Tebot Bach. She's published poems, essays, and articles in more than 150 journals, magazines, and newspapers, including *Prairie Schooner, Poet Lore, Margie, Nimrod, The Laurel Review*, and *Ploughshares*, and given more than 150 writing workshops, including the San Miguel Writers' Conference, Centrum, and the Marine and Science

Technology Center. Finishing Line Press published her chapbook *Other Voices*; Prentice Hall published *Student Reflection Journal for Student Success*. A former journalist, she taught writing, media, and diversity/globalism classes at Highline College for twenty-seven years and at Shanghai Jiao Tong University in 2002, 2008, 2010, and 2012 through an exchange between Highline and Jiao Tong. A book of writing exercises is forthcoming from Two Sylvias Press in 2018. Last week, a dragonfly landed and stayed on her right arm for several minutes—a sign of good luck.

ANGELA LOCKE is a writer and teacher who spends winters in Upstate New York and looks forward to the June gloom of early summer in Santa Barbara. In either place, she is accompanied by her go-to girl, Emma, a heeler-pit bull mix.

PERIE LONGO, Poet Laureate Emerita (2007-2009) of Santa Barbara, has published four books of poetry: *Milking the Earth, The Privacy of Wind, With Nothing Behind but Sky: A Journey Through Grief,* and most recently, *Baggage Claim* (2014). Nominated for three Pushcart Prizes, her work has appeared in numerous journals, including *Askew, Atlanta Review, Connecticut Review, International Poetry Review, Levure litteraire, Live Encounters, Miramar, Nimrod, Paterson Literary Review, Poet Lore, Prairie Schooner, Quercus Review, Rattle, Solo,* and *South Carolina Review.* She has been on the staff of the annual Santa Barbara Writers Conference since 1984, and every summer leads a two-day poetry workshop. She taught with California-Poets-in-the-Schools from 1985-2014, teaches poetry privately, and is Poetry Chair for the Nuclear Age Peace Foundation. As a psychotherapist, she integrates poetry for healing. In 2005 she was invited to speak at the University of Kuwait on Poetry as a way to Peace.

EILEEN MALONE'S poetry has been published in more than 500 literary journals and anthologies, a significant amount of which have earned awards, including three Pushcart nominations.

Her award-winning collection, *Letters with Taloned Claws*, was published by Poets Corner Press (Sacramento) and her book, *I Should Have Given Them Water*, was published by Ragged Sky Press (Princeton).

Leslie Anne Mcilroy won the 1997 Slipstream Poetry Chapbook Prize for *Gravel*, the 2001 Word Press Poetry Prize for her full-length collection *Rare Space*, and the 1997 Chicago Literary Awards. Her second book, *Liquid Like This*, was published by Word Press in 2008, and *Slag*, published by Main Street Rag Publishing Company in December 2014, was runner-up in their 2014 Poetry Book Prize. Leslie's poems appear or are forthcoming in *Bacopa Literary Review* ("Big Bang" won second place for the 2016 Bacopa Literary Review Prize), *Grist*, *Jubilat*, *The Mississippi Review*, *PANK*, *Pearl*, *Poetry Magazine*, the *New Ohio Review*, *The Chiron Review*, and more. She is managing editor of HEArt—Human Equity through Art. Leslie works as a copywriter in Pittsburgh, where she lives with her daughter, Silas.

Missy Michaels lived almost her entire life in Melbourne, Australia, with the exception of two action-packed years in New York City, where she worked as a location scout and studied filmmaking. She wrote and directed several documentary films, and has worked as a freelance writer for the past fifteen years. She attended writing workshops in the United States and Greece with author Cheryl Strayed, who encouraged her to write this essay.

Bernadette Murphy is the author of *Harley and Me: Embracing Risk on the Road to a More Authentic Life* (Counterpoint Press, May 2016). She has published three previous books of narrative nonfiction, including the bestselling *Zen and the Art of Knitting*, is an associate professor in the Creative Writing Department of Antioch University Los Angeles, and a former weekly book critic for the Los Angeles Times. Bernadette-Murphy.com.

MARIANNE PEEL is a poet and a flute-playing vocalist, learning to play ukulele, who is raising four daughters. She shares her life with her partner Scott, whom she met in Istanbul while studying in Turkey. Marianne taught middle and high school English for thirty-two years, and participated in Marge Piercy's Juried Intensive Poetry Workshop in June 2016. She recently won first prize for poetry in the spring 2016 edition of *Gadfly Literary Magazine*, and also won the Pete Edmonds Poetry Prize. Marianne has been published in *Muddy River Review; Silver Birch Press; Persephone's Daughters; Encodings: A Feminist Literary Journal; Write to Heal; Writing for Our Lives: Our Bodies—Hurts, Hungers, Healing; Mother Voices; Metropolitan Woman Magazine; Ophelia's Mom; Jellyfish Whispers; Remembered Arts Journal*, and *Gravel*, among others.

TANIA PRYPUTNIEWICZ, a graduate of the Iowa Writers' Workshop, is a co-founding blogger for Tarot for Two and the author of *November Butterfly* (Saddle Road Press, 2014). Tania's poems have been published or are forthcoming in *A Year in Ink, The Chiron Review, Everyday Haiku Anthology, Nimrod International Journal*, and *Whale Road Review*. She teaches a monthly poetry workshop for San Diego Writers, Ink and lives in Coronado, CA, with her husband, three children, a blue-eyed Husky, and a portly housecat named Luna. taniapryputniewicz.com.

DIANA RAAB, MFA, Ph.D., is a memoirist, poet, blogger, speaker, and award-winning author of nine books. Her work has been published and anthologized in over 500 publications. She holds a Ph.D. in psychology with a research focus on the healing and transformative powers of writing. She blogs for *Psychology Today, PsychAlive, Elephant Journal*, and *The Huffington Post*. She's editor of two anthologies: *Writers and Their Notebooks* and *Writers on the Edge*; two memoirs: *Regina's Closet: Finding My Grandmother's Secret Journal* and *Healing with Words: A Writer's Cancer Journey*, and four poetry collections, including *Lust*. Much of her inspiration comes from diarist and writer, Anaïs Nin. Her latest book is *Writing for*

Bliss: A Seven-Step Program for Telling Your Story and Transforming Your Life (September 2017). dianaraab.com

DIANE RAPTOSH's fourth book of poetry, *American Amnesiac* (Etruscan Press), was long-listed for the 2013 National Book Award and was a finalist for the Housatonic Book Award. The recipient of three fellowships in literature from the Idaho Commission on the Arts, she served as the Boise Poet Laureate (2013) as well as the Idaho Writer-in-Residence (2013-2016), the highest literary honor in the state. Her poems have appeared in numerous literary journals and anthologies in the United States and Canada. A highly active ambassador for poetry, she has given poetry workshops everywhere from riverbanks to maximum-security prisons. She teaches creative writing and runs the program in Criminal Justice/Prison Studies at The College of Idaho. Her most recent collection of poems, *Human Directional*, was released by Etruscan Press in fall 2016. dianeraptosh.com

LISA RIZZO is the author of *Always a Blue House* (Saddle Road Press, 2016) and *In the Poem an Ocean,* a chapbook (Big Table Publishing, 2011). Her work also has appeared in such journals and anthologies as *13th Moon, Calyx Journal, Naugatuck River Review,* and *Everyday Haiku* (Wandering Muse Press). Two of her poems received first and second place prizes in the 2011 Maggi H. Meyer Poetry Prize competition. Living in the San Francisco Bay Area, Lisa works as an instructional coach helping teachers improve their reading and writing instruction. This is her first nonfiction publication. lisarizzopoetry.com

BARBARA ROCKMAN teaches poetry at Santa Fe Community College, leads private writing workshops in New Mexico, and brings poetry to victims of domestic violence as Workshop Coordinator for Wingspan Poetry Project. She frequently collaborates with artists in word and image installations. Her poems appear widely in journals and anthologies and have been nominated for three Pushcart

Prizes and awarded the Southwest Writers Prize and Baskerville Publishers Award. Her collection, *Sting and Nest*, received the New Mexico-Arizona Book Award and the National Press Women Book Prize. She earned her MFA from Vermont College of Fine Arts and lives in Santa Fe, New Mexico.

MINDELA RUBY is the author of the novel *Mosh It Up* (2014). Her short works have appeared in or are forthcoming in *Rivet*, *WomanArts Quarterly*, *East Bay Review*, *Literary Mama*, and elsewhere. In 2016 her poems were nominated for a Pushcart Prize and the *Sundress Best of the Net Anthology*. She holds a Ph.D. from the University of California.

Born and raised in New England, BECKY DENNISON SAKELLARIOU has lived most of her adult life in Greece. She now divides her time between New Hampshire and the island of Euboia, north of Athens. A teacher, writer/editor and counselor, Becky has published poetry in many journals, most recently in *White Pelican Review*, *Comstock Review*, *Persimmon Tree*, and *Common Ground Review*. A winner in several poetry contests and nominated for the Pushcart Poetry Anthology twice, she won first prize in the 2005 Blue Light Press Chapbook Contest for *The Importance of Bone*. In 2010, her first full-length book, *Earth Listening*, was chosen by Hobblebush Books in Brookline, NH, as the second in its Granite State Poetry Series. In 2014, Becky put out a second chapbook, *What Shall I Cry?*, with Finishing Line Press, and another in 2015, *Gathering the Soft*, with Passager Press. Her latest, *No Foothold in this Geography*, with Blue Light Press, is available on Amazon. beckysakellariou.com.

CATHIE SANDSTROM's work has appeared in Ploughshares, The Southern Review, Lyric, Comstock Review, Cider Press Review, and Ekphrasis, among others. Her work can be read in the anthology *Wide Awake: Poets of Los Angeles and Beyond*, and *Master Class: The Poetry Mystique*. She was a finalist in the Poets & Writers' California

Writers Exchange, and her chapbook *A Non-Believer's Book of Hours* won honorable mention at *The Comstock Review*. Her poem, "You, Again" is in the artists' book collection at the Getty Museum in Los Angeles and at the University of Southern California.

MARIANNE TAYLOR received the Allen Ginsberg Award, the Helen A. Quade Award, and an *Iowa Woman* Poetry Prize. Her manuscript, *Salt Water, Iowa*, has been a finalist in a half-dozen contests. Her poetry appears widely in anthologies and national journals such as *Nimrod International, North American Review, Alaska Quarterly* and *Alehouse*. She also writes and directs plays, teaches literature and creative writing at Kirkwood Community College, and recently served on the Mount Vernon, IA, City Council.

RUTH THOMPSON's "fierce, gorgeous, sensual" poems of earth-as-body and body-as-earth have been collected in three books of poetry: *Crazing; Woman With Crows;* and *Here Along Cazenovia Creek*. Her work has won *New Millennium Writings, Chautauqua,* and *Tupelo Quarterly* awards. It has appeared in *bosque, Poetry Flash, Sow's Ear Poetry Review, Chautauqua, Potomac Review, Naugatuck River Review, Poetry Daily,* and has been choreographed by Shizuno Nasu and Jennifer Eng. Ruth received a BA from Stanford and a doctorate in English from Indiana University. She teaches poetry, meditation, and writing from the body workshops ("Body Speaking"), and is editor of a small literary press in Hilo, Hawai'i. ruththompson.net

CARINE TOPAL, a transplanted New Yorker, lives in the Southern California desert. Her work has appeared in numerous journals and anthologies such as *The Best of the Prose Poem, Scrivener Creative Review, Caliban, Greensboro Review, Iron Horse Literary Review,* and many others. She was nominated for a Pushcart Prize in 2004, and was awarded residency at Hedgebrook, and a fellowship to study in St. Petersburg, Russia in 2005. She won the 2007 Robert G. Cohn Prose Poetry Award from California Arts and Letters, from which a special edition chapbook, *Bed of Want*, was published. Her 3rd collection of poetry, *In the Heaven of Never Before*, was published in December, 2008, by Moon Tide Press. In the same year she was honored with the Excellence in Arts Award from the City of Torrance, California. In 2015 Carine won the Briar Cliff Review Poetry Contest, was nominated, once again, for a Pushcart Prize, and her new poetry collection, *Tattooed*, won the Palettes and Quills 4th Biennial Chapbook Contest. She teaches poetry and memoir in the Palm Springs and Los Angeles areas.

DAVI WALDERS' poetry and prose have appeared in more than 200 anthologies and journals. Her collection on women's resistance during WWII, *Women Against Tyranny: Poems of Resistance During the Holocaust*, was published by Clemson University Press. Other collections include *Using Poetry in Therapeutic Settings*, published by The Vital Signs Poetry Project at NIH and its Children's Inn. She developed the Vital Signs Project at NIH in Bethesda, MD, which was funded by The Witter Bynner Foundation for Poetry and for which she received Hadassah of Greater Washington's Myrtle Wreath Award. Other awards include a Maryland Artist Grant in Poetry, an Alden B. Dow Creativity Fellowship, and fellowships at Virginia Center for the Creative Arts, Ragdale, Hebrew Union College in Cincinnati, and elsewhere. Her work has been read by Garrison Keillor on Writer's Almanac, nominated for Pushcart Prizes, and choreographed and performed in NYC, Michigan, Cleveland, and elsewhere.

PHYLLIS WAX writes in Milwaukee on a bluff overlooking Lake Michigan. Her poetry has appeared in *Ars Medica, Naugatuck River Review, Verse Wisconsin, Mobius: The Journal of Social Change, Out of Line* and *The New Verse News*, as well as many other journals and anthologies, both print and online. Three of her poems are included in *The Widows' Handbook: Poetic Reflections on Grief and Survival* (Kent State University Press.) She participated in *Threaded Metaphors: Text and Textiles*, collaborations between six poets and six fiber artists. Her work has been nominated for a Pushcart Prize. Phyllis can be reached at poetwax38@gmail.com

SARAH BROWN WEITZMAN has been published in hundreds of journals and anthologies, including *Rosebud, The New Ohio Review, Poet & Critic, The North American Review, Rattle, Mid-American Review, Poet Lore, Spillway,* and many others. Sarah received a fellowship from the National Endowment for the Arts. A departure from poetry, her fourth book, *Herman and the Ice Witch,* is a children's novel published by Main Street Rag.

JULIE WENGLINSKI was born in St. Louis and spent many years growing up in central Florida, where her father worked for the space program. After receiving a biology degree in 1975 in Boca Raton, Julie moved to Richmond, VA, and worked for thirty years in IT. After retirement, she married for the first time at the age of fifty-seven and began taking writing classes through the Virginia Museum of Fine Arts. She has published both poems and flash fiction.

LORI WHITE's recent essays have appeared in *Hobart, Mud Season Review, The Boiler,* and *The Nervous Breakdown* (thenervousbreakdown. com). Her short story, "Gambling One Ridge Away," won first place in the 2013 Press 53 Open Award for Flash Fiction. She teaches English composition at Los Angeles Pierce College.

BRENDA YATES grew up on military bases. After living in Tennessee, Delaware, Florida, Michigan, Massachusetts, Japan and Hawaii, she settled first in Boston, then Los Angeles. Her poems have appeared in numerous journals and anthologies including *Mississippi Review, City of the Big Shoulders: An Anthology of Chicago Poetry (University of Iowa Press)* and *The Southern Poetry Anthology, Volume VI: Tennessee (Texas Review Press).* She is a Pushcart nominee and recipient of the Beyond Baroque Literary Arts Center Poetry Prize, a Patricia Bibby Prize, and was a finalist in the Robinson Jeffers Tor House Poetry Contest. Her collection, *Bodily Knowledge,* was published by Tebot Bach in 2015.

CPSIA information can be obtained
at www.ICGtesting.com
Printed in the USA
FSHW01n0906180918
52254FS